Charles Popper

The Impulsive Personality

UNDERSTANDING PEOPLE WITH DESTRUCTIVE CHARACTER DISORDERS

The Impulsive Personality

UNDERSTANDING PEOPLE WITH DESTRUCTIVE CHARACTER DISORDERS

Howard Wishnie, M.D.

Cambridge Hospital
Harvard Medical School

Plenum Press · New York and London

Library of Congress Cataloging in Publication Data

Wishnie, Howard
  The impulsive personality.

  Includes index.
  1. Personality, Disorders of. 2. Impulse. 3. Narcotic addicts. 4. Criminal psychology.
5. Sociopathic personality. 6. Psychotherapy. I. Title. [DNLM: 1. Antisocial personality. 2. Compulsive behavior. WM210 W814]
RC554.W57   616.8'58   77-23464
ISBN 0-306-30973-4

© 1977 Plenum Press, New York
A Division of Plenum Publishing Corporation
227 West 17th Street, New York, N.Y. 10011

Printed in the United States of America

To the memory of
ELVIN V. SEMRAD,
a man who taught generations of
therapists that humanism and compassion are the
cornerstones of psychotherapy

Preface

I began this book with two purposes. One goal was to present clinical information to support the belief that many of society's allegedly untreatable people could be helped to change their destructive patterns of living. A second purpose was to present a clear and simple primer for two groups of workers in the field.

Most treatment institutions depend upon the services of nurses, aides, guards, and corrections officers. These people, who are the least prepared, do the bulk of the treatment. Because impulsive people learn much from their daily interactions outside of formal therapy, the understanding and the training of this "front-line" working staff are crucial. These staff members may find the second part of the book more helpful because of its use of clinical examples and techniques.

The other group for whom this book is written includes those who are beginning in the mental health or corrections field. The concept of useful treatment of impulse-ridden people has only begun to be introduced into professional training programs. The assumption that these individuals were untreatable has kept many professionals at the fringes of this field. For this reason, I hope that the book will find its way into the hands of psychiatric residents, psychologists, social workers, nurses, probation officers, prison guards, youth workers, policemen, judges, etc.

The book is divided into two sections. The first four chapters deal with my beliefs, experiences, and theoretical understandings. The rest of the book provides a series of practical experiences and concepts. The material does not attempt to provide a specific answer, only an approach that can be combined with other ideas to develop treatment methods.

HOWARD WISHNIE

Cambridge

Acknowledgments

The understanding and organization of any material is an effort that draws upon the experience of many people. In this effort, I am indebted to many people.

There are, first of all, the many patients and staff members at various institutions from whom I have learned. They provided the experiences that forced me to reexamine old beliefs in order to achieve different perspectives.

Five teachers in my early training deserve special thanks from me and many other students: Drs. Elvin Semrad, Jack Ewalt, Elizabeth Zetzel, John MacKenzie, and Irene Briggin. These teachers, through their direct supervision and writings, sensitized me to the pain inherent in one's early development and later behavior. My learning experience with these five doctors forms the underpinning for this work.

As my interests shifted toward impulsive people, three other teachers were a consistent help and stimulus. Drs. George Vaillant, Norman Zinberg, and Arnold M. Ludwig are already known for their clear thinking in the area of addiction and impulse disorders. They constantly challenged me to rethink my premises and refine my ideas.

The organization of this book received much of its impetus for completion from Mrs. Evelyn Stone, whose encouragement was of immeasurable value.

Dr. Richard Cowan was both companion and support throughout my Lexington experience, a burden he shared with Mr. Larry Welding and Mrs. Emily Cummings. Together we four formed a nuclear group that tried to work for change when others said it was impossible.

During all of this, my wife has sustained and reassured me. Her belief in my capacity to understand and to make sense of my experience allowed me to pursue the task of writing. She, and the children, tolerated the days and weekends when I wrote and was not with them.

H.W.

Contents

Introduction

The intent of this book is to assist the individual who chooses to work with impulsive people in the formulation of a coherent approach to treatment. National and international awareness of the problems caused by characteristically impulsive people is growing. Broad measures of their presence are seen in the increasing crime rate, escalating drug abuse, widespread alcoholism, and the necessity to develop more hospital space for nonpsychotic, impulse-ridden individuals.

The characteristics of these impulsive people will be briefly mentioned here and defined more clearly in the text that follows.

People with impulsive character problems, when viewed over a span of time, seem to be living in a state of constant but stable chaos. They appear to be intensely involved in their momentary activities and to possess little perspective about the future consequences of their current behavior. Similarities to past situations are ignored or hostilely disregarded; they seem to be reacting only to the current problem. These are people who live only in the present, who seem to view their lives as taking a steady and irrevocable downhill course in which their only possible choice of action is to diminish the rate of decline to ultimate destruction.

With this perspective about time and their ultimate destiny, the impulsive speak of themselves as victims of fate, society, social injustice, etc. They have given up in terms of affecting their own lives. They use this sense of powerlessness to justify the attitude of living for the moment. With a desperate, angry quality, they pursue and demand some momentary satisfaction, which is always less gratifying than they had wished. Their chronic anger and desperation are seen in their lashing-out at friends, family, and society.

Any behavior is justified because they have been victimized from the beginning. In their behavior they demonstrate a rejection of any societal norms and restraints. It is their right to behave as they please, since they were given less than others. Behavior becomes the key factor in understanding such people. Many are skillful and gifted in terms of speech and rationalization. They can be beguiling; yet, their behavior, which is inconsistent over time, belies their words. Thus, treatment will rely more upon observations of behavior than upon verbal interactions, explanations, promises, etc.

These individuals show a poor capacity to take care of themselves and little ability to develop lasting and satisfying relationships with others. Impulse-ridden people may verbally express great concern for the people in their lives but in actuality show little capacity to care for and respond to their needs. Over a period of time, one frequently observes a steady flow of changing people. The impulsive individual ostensibly cares a great deal for these people, but there is little evidence of this care. Their lives may involve many changing relationships or a shunning of others. Essentially their anger and futility about themselves interferes with a capacity to relate to others as real people. The quality of their relationships has a more cardboard or plastic nature. The needs, feelings, and wishes of others are seen as unreal and as an intrusion. It is as if the person with an impulsive personality views himself as the principal actor on a stage, with all other people as a supporting cast. We see this in its most extreme form in senseless acts of violence and brutality wherein the perpetrator has no concern or remorse for the victim. Yet, such an individual can assume an attitude of grief or remorse if he feels it will achieve a desired effect.

Treatment approaches to working with impulsive people range from punitive and repressive to liberal and unstructured. One senses a competitiveness among treatment modalities as to which approach is "right" and represents "the answer." Rather than espouse a particular treatment, I have attempted to develop a logical approach to treatment design. Basic to such an approach is an understanding of the origin and development of impulsive character traits and their protective (defensive) function in the individual's past and current life. With this developmental understanding in mind, I go on to observe these traits in the treatment situation.

Impulsive people graphically relive their internal struggles in the arena of interpersonal relationships. This occurs in any setting, be it marriage, job, prison, hospital, clinic, etc. They come with a prepared script into which they fit the new actors. Thus, one is not seen as an individual but as a new, slightly different version of a familiar character. Part of the treatment requires the identification of these characters and the definition of their roles in the patient's life.

Currently, one of the best places for learning about impulsive character pathology is in the treatment of drug addicts. The widespread abuse of drugs has led to the development of many treatment settings with vastly different approaches, all of which seem to be struggling with the same kind of impulsive, self-destructive behavior. It is not that drug abusers represent a discrete diagnostic entity; they are just more accessible than incarcerated criminals. The abuse of drugs is one of a series of maladaptive maneuvers that the individual develops to cope with specific internal feelings of desperation and anger. Because these maneuvers are poorly conceived and organized, one sees a chaotic moving-about from one impulsive stance to another. Thus, the individual seen in the drug clinic today may appear in the psychiatric ward in three months for treatment of a depression; six months later, one may find him jailed for robbery and assault. Understanding the defensive need for this behavior leads to the development of rational treatment approaches that focus less upon the most recent symptomatic manifestation and more upon the underlying motivation. *It is the underlying char-*

acter that must change, or one is constantly looking for treatment of the newest manifestation.

The reader will note that I have borrowed from many schools of psychology and sociology. No one theory or approach contains all of the necessary understandings, yet all seem to contribute to a better understanding and treatment of impulsive character pathology. The sophisticated reader who may legitimately object to this simplified, synthetic approach should bear in mind that the book is written in a simple manner to convey an understanding of some of the basic treatment problems encountered in this work. It is a beginner's book written by a beginner, avoiding jargon and technical shorthand so that both the high school graduate and the advanced student will be able to read and understand it.

The Author's Premises

Attempts to write about the theory and treatment of any emotional dysfunction necessitate the author's introduction of his and the patient's beliefs. Rather than having these premises appear in the text, it is best to enumerate them at the outset so that the reader can weigh their influence upon a particular issue.

The fact that this book is written to assist the patient (addict, criminal, etc.) and his would-be counselor (therapist) implies several such beliefs.

Character Traits Can Change!

The patient will repeatedly try to seduce the therapist into confirming his belief that, he, the patient, is unchangeable. ("Aw, c'mon, Doc, what do you expect from a junkie?" "You know I'm like that.") The constant attempt on the part of the patient to get the therapist to agree to the immutable quality of the patient's character plays a key role in treatment.

Treatment Is a Means of Changing Character

Treatment involves a relationship between two or more people. At least one person is defined as a patient or client and at least one person is defined as a counselor or therapist. The effectiveness of any treatment method depends upon the character of the relationship between the patient and therapist. This basic human relationship requires close attention, no matter what the treatment method may be. Thus, the therapist must be aware of and examine his own beliefs, attitudes, responses, feelings, expectations, and behavior with regard to the patient. He must observe the same factors in the patient. Casually conducted treatments that consider high ideals and good intentions as an adequate safeguard against error are stupid and naive. Such nonsensical approaches have no place in serious treatment. Therapist and patient are obligated to assess themselves and their work carefully.

For example, in a psychiatric treatment setting, a new therapist insisted upon wearing antiwar buttons and armbands. Other staff felt that these statements of political belief could potentially interfere with the basic work of the treatment unit, since patients of many political beliefs came to the unit. The issue came up at a patient–staff meeting where a previously silent schizophrenic patient spoke up and said, "This is my third time in the hospital. I'm very confused. They tell me I have schizophrenia. I don't know what that is. I come here for help; I don't want to think about your politics."

In a second situation, a female staff member came to work braless in revealing clothes. One patient, a secretly impotent depressed young man, consistently argued with her. He assumed a bravado stance of provocative superiority and one day made a pass at her. Later discussion revealed that he felt shamed and humiliated at the idea of needing help from anyone, much less a woman. Being closeted in a small room with a young woman who unthinkingly taunted him with her body made it difficult for him to speak of his impotence, rage, and neediness.

While no treatment can avoid the introduction of personal beliefs, the obligation is to limit them where possible and assess their impact where they are present.

Treatment and the Needs of the Individual

Many people who characteristically behave in an impulsive and destructive manner (criminals, alcoholics, addicts, habitually assaultive individuals, impulse-ridden borderline patients, etc.) are treatable with specifically designed psychotherapies. These treatment approaches consist of a combination of ideas that emerge from the psychodynamic, psychoanalytic, behavioral, and transactional analytic schools of thought. At times, drug therapies may be necessary adjuncts before the psychotherapies can be useful.

The failure of many previous treatment attempts can be traced to a misapplication of psychiatric principles developed for the treatment of non-impulse-ridden individuals. The neurotic patient seeks consultation because he perceives a problem: "Doctor, I do well at work or with my friends, but when I call a girl for a date I stammer and fumble," or "I got a B on an exam and it felt like an F." The patient identifies an issue that is a problem for himself. He sees the therapist as a potential helper through the exchange of ideas and the review of past experiences. By and large, he manages his life in an adequate fashion that does not force others to watch over him.

The impulse-ridden person is frequently brought to the treatment setting under duress: "My probation officer says I have to see you," "My lawyer said it would be good to see a drug counselor before I go to court," "It's this place or jail, I had to choose." Unlike the neurotic individual, who may overvalue the therapist, the impulse-ridden person is more likely to devalue the therapist, denying that there's a problem in the way he lives: "Look, I don't need a shrink. If they made drugs legal, I'd be O.K. That's the problem, so what good are you, anyhow?" There is no discrete problem. The individual is a victim of an unfair system. As proof, wasn't he forced to see you? To sit with such a person and passively inquire about his feelings and memories without addressing his role in his current predicament would be foolish. Although his behavior is motivated by dynamic issues similar to those of the more neurotic individual, initial work in therapy must address the impact of behavior and the need for modulation of the expression of feeling. Subsequent work moves in the direction of identifying the individual problems in terms of his interpersonal behavior and his role in these problems. Only later, when the individual is responsible for his own behavior and sees how he creates interpersonal problems, will this naturally lead to an understanding of the intrapsychic conflicts that are more neurotic in origin. Thus, early treatment work may focus more upon behavior, limits, expectations, goals, and interpersonal observations. The planning of treatment requires the therapist to assess these intrapsychic conflicts and adapt his treatment accordingly. To attempt analysis or psychotherapy with someone who does not assume responsibility for his own behavior, nor value his own words and thoughts as an honest representation of his perception of himself, is a contradiction of the principle of these two modalities.

Society's Unreasonable Expectations

Although there is a continued national concern with the effect of drug usage upon the individual and society, there is an increasing sense of disillusionment and futility about our attempts to cope with this problem. As with other social experiments, experience has shown that many individuals and national policy-planning groups have rushed to develop large-scale solutions for social ills before they have adequately studied and understood the complexity of the problem (prohibition to cure alcoholism, punitive jails to rehabilitate criminals, legislative programs to end poverty). Drug abuse has been no exception to this approach. There is an apparent belief that the expenditure of large sums of money and the involvement of great numbers of people will somehow overwhelm the issue of drug abuse by sheer force. Unfortunately, when such massive approaches do not result in equally impressive results, the creators of such programs, as well as the workers and the patients, tend to become disillusioned and bitter. As a result of such disillusionment, small successes as well as potentially useful knowledge are dismissed as inadequate, and the patient (addict, criminal) is then deemed untreatable and suitable only for chronic confinement. Many prisons and state and VA hospitals illustrate this. It is as if society is rejecting these persons who disabuse us of our beliefs about rapid social and personal change. Until we are willing to consider the origins of our social ills and involve ourselves in long-term evolutionary programs, we will continue to punish those who teach us that we are not smart enough nor powerful enough to change a person's character in a brief span of time.

For those who doubt the validity of this, there is the current attempt to close state hospitals and return mental patients to their home communities. A basically sound and humane goal may fail because the home communities have been poorly prepared and many patients are existing under more harsh conditions than those that prevailed in the state hospitals. It is only a matter of time before there will be a reopening of these institutions. Prison reform and furlough programs are under pressure of curtailment or dissolution. Noble ideas are discredited because of inadequate planning and implementation. Thus, an idea that is valid may be put aside to the detriment of all.

When the initial plans fail to deal with numerous important factors, little effort is subsequently spent analyzing the reasons for successes or failures or supporting the positive programs that do emerge. There is an all-or-nothing quality to our social planning. Few programs take into account the necessity for long-term planning and evaluation in terms of years and decades. Although we should like the quality of human life to improve rapidly, the process of substantive change requires time. To have expected or publicly stated that the War on Poverty or the Great Society would relieve the social ills of this country in a few years was ridiculous!

We have already seen a similar process of unrealistic expectations developing in persons who have been working with drug addicts. Admittedly, there is no single, effective cure for drug addiction; there is no single addict type. One hears people passionately proclaim that their techniques—methadone, religion, self-help, etc.—represent *the* answer and should be adhered to at the exclusion of all others. The addict has come to use drugs for a variety of reasons. He has chosen them as a partial solution to personal problems. He has suffered from a host of personal difficulties that have resulted in the formation of character deficits before he turned to the narcotic–analgesic solution.

While it seems to be true that the addict's drug use must be stopped before effective treatment can begin, the *preexisting character problems must be dealt with or the drug use will begin anew!*

Social Pressures and Impulsive Behavior

While we are all subject to various group and cultural pressures, all too often these pressures are used to mask the individual's role (choice) in his own behavior. Treatment modalities that foster a negative group identity and view the individual *solely* as the victim of social oppression do a disservice to the individual. They contribute to the hopelessness of the individual and lead to desperate actions. If social oppression were the major reason for self-destructive and impulsive behavior, how would one explain that the great majority of socially oppressed individuals are not impulsively self-destructive?

Individuals are better served by treatment methods that help them to see their own role in the development of their problems. We are less overwhelmed when contending with problems of our own making than when contending with those of a more global nature.

As an example of the destructive effect of developing an awareness of a negative group identity, one can see the emergence of militant homosexuality. Gay liberation is legitimately moving forward in diminishing the stigma and isolation of homosexuality, while affirming the genuine legal and social rights of homosexuals. At the same time, however, it tends to cloud over the basic unhappiness and limitations of relationships that homosexuals experience. These limitations are not based upon societal pressures but develop out of the dynamics of homosexuality. As a result, many homosexuals view their personal unhappiness as a result of society's pressure. They overlook the more important internal issues and waste years before realizing that they need to resolve their personal problems.

Similarly, a black criminal may have his criminality supported as an understandable expression of his social oppression as a black rather than as a personal response to internal feelings. Because so many groups and therapists want to use his behavior to prove the existence of a general social symptom, no one listens to him as an individual.

Thus, in developing treatment programs one needs to keep a perspective upon the relative influence of group and cultural issues versus personal and individual issues. This approach runs counter to the prevailing trends that view any deviant behavior as a result of cultural pressures for which the individual has little responsibility. Effective treatment requires this balanced perspective. Society will change when the individuals within it change themselves.

Staff Attitude and Impulsive Behavior

As an outgrowth of the previous issues, it is clear that the attitudes of treatment staff at an institution may tend to promote or diminish the continuation of impulsive behavior. Staff-supported continuation of impulsive behavior may occur when treatment concepts are vague or useless and the staff's disillusionment is not addressed. The work of any individual therapist can be seriously undermined by inconsistencies in the approaches of the rest of the treatment staff. The more intensive the treatment approach, the greater the necessity for staff members to evaluate and discuss their own attitudes and behavior. Inconsistent behavior by an administrator or an indirectly involved staff member can become fertile ground for the self-doubts and hopelessness of the patient. As is true of patients, staff behavior can be a more clear-cut indicator of attitude than their words. Observations that the staff are personally sloppy and haphazard, have little regard for each other, and fail to attend scheduled meetings can undercut the best-formulated plans.

This does not mean that the staff must agree on every issue. It does mean that the staff must have respectful means of *openly* disagreeing about issues, as well as an adequate degree of self- and mutual respect. Members of the staff act as role models for a highly suspicious and skeptical group of patients who are looking for ways to discount the validity of treatment methods. Treatment with an energetic staff that demonstrates the process of open disagreement and conflict resolution is more effective than treatment in the setting of an outwardly compliant staff that blindly follows the rules and by its own passivity undermines its own work.

Drug Addiction as a Manifestation of Impulsive Behavior

I view much of drug addiction as one phase of ongoing impulsive character pathology. In shifting the reader's attention to drug abuse, I focus upon the general principles of impulsive and self-destructive character dysfunction as they appear at the time of drug abuse. The same individual seen at a later date might show similar traits under a different label. In other words, these traits should not be viewed as solely those of drug addicts.

At this time, there is a tendency to view impulsive individuals in terms of narrowly defined categories that are based upon the most apparent or troubling current symptoms. An example illustrates this problem:

Esteban made a number of appearances in various segments of a community treatment program over a 2½ year period. He was first seen during a psychiatric hospitalization for a suicide attempt and depression following the breakup of his marriage. He had a prior history of alcohol and drug abuse and juvenile delinquency, as well as a discharge from the army for malingering. After several days on the ward, he was more energetic in his behavior, his speech was clear, and he seemed comfortable and no longer depressed. He became irritable if asked about the recent or remote past, blamed his ex-wife for his problems, and denied that alcohol or drug abuse would be problems again. His behavior was labile. He could rapidly shift from happy-go-lucky to menacingly angry or expansively happy over a period of an hour. These changes occurred in response to the extent to which he was asked to deal with his own behavior. He was discharged against advice and was seen as having an impulsive character disorder. Several weeks later, he was arrested for car theft, breaking and entry, and assault. To the police, he was primarily a small-time criminal. While on probation, he had himself admitted to an inpatient drug unit for detoxification from barbiturates. After several days and several fights, he was discharged as a chronic drug abuser. Several months later, he was admitted to the alcohol detoxification unit at the same mental health center, where he was seen as being primarily an alcoholic. Upon discharge, he went to jail for 6 months and returned to the system, where he resurfaced several times in the mental health and penal systems. After 2½ years, he was dead of an overdose.

None of us had effectively grappled with his destructive character problem. During the 2½ years he was known to us, there had been a number of discussions among the staff of the various units. Basically, these discussions boiled down to disagreements as to whether he was really an addict, or an alcoholic, or an impulsive character, or a chronic criminal, or maybe schizophrenic. Which diagnosis best defined him? Each unit, set up with its own narrow expertise, tended to see greater merit in its own diagnostic criteria. We had no useful clinical model of conceptualizing this individual in an overall manner that took into account his varying symptom manifestations.

Another view of this problem comes from data gathered at the former Clinical Research Center for drug addicts at Lexington, Kentucky. Histories of 70 consecutively admitted patients showed the following patterns: cigarette smoking and experimentation with alcohol by age 10–12; weekend binges by age 15; barbiturate abuse and delinquent behavior by age 17; heroin addiction and criminal behavior by age 19; imprisonment by age 24. Older addicts, who were fewer in number at Lexington, seemed to stabilize in their addiction by age 35–40, requiring a small, set amount of drug each day. Other older addicts tended to work at regular jobs or a regular criminal activity by age 40 and used alcohol and drugs in small amounts. The smallness of the number of older addicts was accounted for in several ways. A number were dead. Others were primarily redefined as criminals and were incarcerated. Some had stabilized in the community as noted. Perhaps others had found different ways to manifest their underlying character problems. Maybe some had resolved their personal issues and developed satisfying lives. Whatever their mode of behavior, these men showed a poor ability to develop lasting relationships in which they did not devalue and punish the people with whom they were involved.

Viewed at a particular time, these men would most likely be labeled with some descriptive term based upon their most visible current problem. *It is this tendency to define the problem by the most pronounced current symptom that interferes with accurate diagnosis and treatment.* In later chapters, I deal with this problem by developing a more integrated concept of impulsive character pathology that takes into account the shifting manifestations.

Specific Premises about Drug-Addicted Impulsive Individuals

The following discussion relates to my biases about impulsive individuals for whom drug abuse is a primary manifestation of their character pathology.

1. If there were a painless way of stopping drug use while

maintaining the comfortable state that the addict experiences while on drugs, he would then probably be inclined toward stopping. It is a fact that, in spite of their drawbacks, the drugs HELP the addict to function and deal with the painful internal feelings that he otherwise finds unbearable. Until he is assured by experience that he will be able to avoid his own sense of emptiness and failure, he will not be willing to give up his drug dependence. The statistics of the U.S. Public Health Service hospitals at Forth Worth, Texas, and Lexington, Kentucky, show that the vast majority of those who stayed for the initial treatment phase of the programs available under the Narcotic Addict Rehabilitation Act of 1966 did so as an alternative to trial or serving a jail sentence. Similarly, the U.S. Army had to make its program of voluntary treatment mandatory, because the number of volunteers was significantly lower than the number of addicted individuals.

The fact that large numbers of addicts seek methadone on the street supports this premise. Methadone is a synthetic narcotic that initially holds out the promise of a cheap and readily accessible source of analgesia. Thus, the addict's reason for seeking it is frequently to cheapen his habit, to relieve family pressure or court pressure, or to provide a baseline of relief of discomfort to which other drugs can be added. His basic *initial* goal is not to alter his way of life but to get immediate relief from pressure. Those people who successfully use methadone maintenance in the process of giving up all drugs, including methadone, do so in the context of programs that provide other interpersonal experiences that aid in character change.

2. There is no single addict[1] type. Most addicts suffer from a variety of character disorders. Underlying these is a sense of personal hopelessness, which the addict avoids through the use of external excitement or narcotics. Thus, he either distracts himself through dangerous activities or doses himself into a transient, bland, thoughtless, and trouble-free state of mind. He

[1] The individual who uses drugs for a brief period during adolescence or a crisis is not the person discussed here. The people herein referred to as addicts are those individuals who consistently use drugs over a long period of time without remission.

does not believe that he can really be effective in changing and influencing his own life.

Contrary to common belief, the opiate drugs do not provide a euphoric, fantasy-filled, and exciting state of mind. Instead, they leave the user withdrawn, empty, trouble-free. The state is more akin to the after-feeding drowsiness of an infant than to the exciting and dramatic feeling often described in the popular press. The "rush" is a brief sensation lasting less than a minute at the onset of injection of the drug.

3. Peer-group pressure and "kicks" are overvalued reasons for the use of drugs. If one is seeking a general reason for drug abuse, I would suggest inadequate family structure and support in early years. When questioned about initial abuse of drugs, many people state that they did it for "kicks" or "to be part of the group." These superficial responses discount the individual decision based upon a personal sense of hopelessness. The following dialogue between C., a 19-year-old addict who has been using drugs for 4 years, and his doctor elucidates this:

> Doctor: "When did you first begin using heroin?"
> Addict: "Oh, I was about 16, Doc."
> "How come?"
> "All the dudes were doing it."
> "All of them?"
> "Well, the guys I wanted to be with, you know, the guys with sharp clothes, the really down dudes."
> "You used it the first time they offered it?"
> (Pause.) "No, I knew it was bad shit and I was afraid, man."
> "Of what?"
> "You know, getting hooked and all, you know. I saw my cousin lose everything when he got strung out on that shit."
> "That held you back initially?"
> "Yeah, I knew it was trouble and it would fuck me up."
> "But there was a time when you finally decided? They didn't hold you down and jab a needle in your arm, did they?"
> "No, man, you know that's stupid. I mean, I might ask

someone to shoot me up but no one would hold me down. I took it."

"Well, then, what changed that made you decide to use it?"

(*Pause.*) "I don't know, I just said fuck it, what the hell. Like it didn't matter."

"What do you mean, it didn't matter?"

"You know, man."

"Make it clear. I really don't know."

"Well, I needed something."

"Yeah? What was missing?"

"How should I know? (*Angrily.*)

"No one else knows the answer but you. Stop dodging around and start looking!"

"Man, it takes me down. Nothing mattered anymore! I just felt bad and decided I'd try it."

"So, what did it do for you?"

"Damn it, it felt good. I just forgot all my problems."

"Problems?"

"Nothing, man, just leave me alone."

Later C. spoke of the sense of futility he had experienced prior to his first use of drugs and his sense of hopelessness. He had come from a severely impoverished home. His parents had separated when he was 5 years old. His father had visited frequently but could not contend with his wife's anger. Both drank and fought. The patient and his brothers were frequently abused by his mother after his father visited. At other times, his mother was described as overly affectionate. Poverty and privation marked his early years. C.'s first use of drugs occurred at age 14, when he found himself repeatedly afraid to talk to girls at dances. "I felt, shit, I couldn't be like the other guys—cool and tough. I don't know why, but I was afraid of these girls. So one night I tried it to make me cool so I could ask this girl, you know." It was his uncertainty and "problems" more than peer-group pressure that influenced his use of drugs.

A general reason for the increase in drug use is the breakdown of family structure. Someone who does not achieve a sense of self-worth through the initial interaction with his parents and siblings will not be able to withstand the turmoil of adolescence. With little hope, and no experience that teaches him that life can be more worthwhile, he attempts to solve his problems and relieve his internal pain through the use of narcotics, alcohol, destructive behavior, etc.

In each instance when an addict has started out talking of kicks, peer-group pressure, and other such reasons for his use of drugs, a much more personal and meaningful answer has been found. Clearly, once drug abuse or destructive behavior has started, peer-group and environmental pressure reinforce the continued use of drugs where there already is a lack of emotional substance and support. The sense of relief provided by the drugs seems to be a more important factor than peer pressure. In fact, many addicts report that drug-using friends initially tried to dissuade them from drug use.

For those who maintain that it is strictly the thrill of the use of drugs, another line of questioning frequently reveals that this, too, is fallacious.

Doctor: "You told us that you were only curious when you began using drugs. If that's the case why did you go back to heroin after the first time?"

Addict: (*Pause. No answer.*)

"You know that narcotic drugs aren't addicting after a single use."

(*Pause.*) "I liked it, man. It made me feel good."

"You liked it better than the way you usually feel?"

"That's right."

"What's the matter with the way you ordinarily feel?"

"Nothing, Doc, I just liked it better."

"That's kind of confusing. Sounds like there was something about the way you ordinarily feel that wasn't as pleasant as being on drugs."

"Yeah, that's true, Doc, there's nothing as good as that high." (*Said with bravado.*)

"Is that the truth?" (*Asked firmly with steady eye contact.*)

"Yeah (*pause*), it is." (*Said sadly, eyes avoiding the interviewer.*)

"You're telling me there's nothing in your life as good as that high? How come?"

(*Pause.*) "I don't know how it got to be that way. Things were always tough, but I did all right. Then, I guess I just gave up."

"Gave up, on what?"

"Everything."

"What?"

"You know, why do I have to say it? (*Pause.*) Me! Me! dammit!"

4. The personal hopelessness of most addicts becomes a specific problem when dealt with in institutions. In prisons and state and other hospitals, as well as in hospitals for the treatment of alcoholism, there is frequently a staff–patient agreement to maintain the status quo. Both share the belief that the goal of positive change and growth is impossible to attain. Staff and patient therefore set up a working system to maintain the most trouble-free existence with the least expenditure of energy by all concerned. Many co-workers and colleagues have said, "You know, these people never change." Patients also say, "You know, I'll never be any different."

A colleague working at a state mental hospital found that the goal of the career staff was to achieve sufficient status to become responsible for a ward. Staff members would then seek to fill the ward with the quietest patients, while trying to exclude disruptive individuals. The staff were not trained for treating mentally ill patients and consequently devised the most workable system for their own comfort. Staff members resented the admission of chaotically disturbed patients who upset the ward. Treatment and clinical improvement were not considered significant possibilities. After several years of working to demonstrate that change and treatment were possible, my friend found the same staff working hard to treat the previously neglected patients.

The patient basically views himself as hopeless and unchangeable. Having no belief in his personal resources, he guards his limited energies for investment in potentially productive activities.

To invest energy in the process of change would be foolish and wasteful. He already knows it is impossible. For this reason, he uses any available energy to maintain the equilibrium that he already possesses. He attempts to make short-term gains without hazarding any loss.

Similarly, the staff frequently preoccupies itself with matters irrelevant to treatment. They may become involved in making gains in the staff rank system: promotions, career advancement, retirement benefits, and the achieving of status. Both staff and patients undermine and at times collaborate in the destruction or removal of anyone or any idea that threatens to disrupt the system, as the following example shows.

A physician entered an institution with a high degree of enthusiasm and energy with regard to treatment. Many of the staff were offended by this and took the attitude "wait and see." Some began placing bets as to when this physician would "burn out" or when "he'll learn that nobody could change the men or the system."

At one point, the physician tried to develop an alternative to discharging individuals who had seriously violated institution rules. He pushed for establishment of a small, separate treatment unit where a man could go for intensive therapy and have a minimum of social diversions. The physician found that, with inadequate staff support, he could not handle this new unit and still carry out his usual duties. In spite of repeated requests for additional assistance, no volunteers emerged. One day, a staff member appeared at his door and smilingly said, "Well, Doc, how come another one of your great ideas failed?" Her satisfaction was evident. The physician asked her about this and inquired if she had been involved in supporting the program. Her answer: "Oh, no! I'm too busy doing *my* job." The physician had made the error of not gaining adequate support within both staff and patient communities before embarking upon a new endeavor. She viewed her job and his job as separate. In spite of discussions with the staff and requests for their participation, they later told him that they had viewed him and his ideas as foreign and threatening. They told him that they wanted him to find out what they knew: no program could be helpful to these men. If he succeeded, their well-rationalized system of behavior would be upset. They would need to reassess their perspectives. The situation did resolve months later, when a greater number of staff members began to share the hope for limited character alteration. Those who could not deal with their own hope-lessness transferred off the unit to work elsewhere in the hospi-tal. The remaining group became more energetic and reported enjoying their work for the first time in years.

In this example as well as that of the state hospital situation, the staff were ordinary individuals whose experience had taught them to view their patients as hopeless and unchangeable. As noted, training and support helped them to review their pre-vious conclusions and invest in their work, with much more satisfying results.

Treatment programs for addicts frequently involve many staff members. Because all staff members participate in the treatment, it is important that all participate in the planning and review of treatment. Staff members who fail to understand the reasoning of a particular treatment approach or who see them-selves and their work as relatively unimportant are less energetic and tend to confuse issues. As a result, they become dissatisfied and undermine the treatment. Where staff members disagree, there should be forums for the resolution of the disagreements. Without the option to discuss and resolve their conflicting views, staff members may actively sabotage treatment.

The presence of open forums for staff discussion does not mean that treatment is a democratic process. Treatment pro-grams and organizations usually place responsibility in the hands of an individual administrator who is ultimately responsible. The administrator may choose to delegate some of his authority but retains his overall responsibility. Most people accept and frankly desire the presence of an individual who represents the ultimate authority. The individual who fulfills this role rarely has to exer-cise his veto power if he is able to explain clearly the reasons for his positions. An arbitrary and capricious administrator who makes decisions without taking his staff into his confidence pro-

motes disrespect, mistrust, and program sabotage (staff acting-
out). It is therefore the responsibility of program directors as
well as the staff to fulfill the role model. Program directors need
to involve themselves in program discussions and to be open to
explanation, questions, and criticism.

   5. Rewards and increased degrees of freedom and responsibility should be based upon the demonstration of a consistent
pattern of behavior, not upon promises or possibilities of change.
Many individuals with destructive character problems are skilled
in presenting themselves to judges, social service agencies,
treatment staff, etc., as people who have significant potential for
growth and change, if only they are given the "right" opportunities. In the evaluation of such an individual, it is important to
question: *What previous evidence has there been that the person
has been seriously interested in change?* One should also wonder: What does he stand to gain now? As a cynic or realist one
must ask: What is it that he really wants or needs? In treatment
settings, repeated assessments of behavior and attitudes are
needed to see if they support a move toward greater degrees of
freedom and responsibility. *If an individual with impulsive character problems is rewarded on the basis of a promise of future
improvement or on the basis of an alleged ability, he will view
this as a successful manipulation and fail to carry through to the
agreed goal.* To be pragmatic, he has received the reward: Why
then bother to expend the effort?

   6. Authors Berne, Harris, and Steiner have described repeating patterns of behavior among people as *games* (interactional patterns), which have scripts (prescribed sequences of
events and outcomes) and roles (definitions of people as acting in
the place of significant persons who are absent). These terms
and perspectives provide a useful and readily understandable
means of identifying recurrent behavior patterns. In this situation, the game is a behavior pattern that aims toward an openly
sought-after goal (acknowledged goal). Of greater consequence,
however, are a series of goals that are not openly acknowledged
and are covert. The covert goals are frequently contradictions of
the acknowledged goal. The following is an example of game behavior:

Elton is a 35-year-old man who entered a drug treatment center after serving 2 years of a 5-year prison sentence. He had been arrested during a store theft. A careful history revealed that he had entered the same warehouse on three previous Saturday nights. On the fourth Saturday night, the police were waiting for him. He later revealed that the store was opposite the police station. In discussing these events and the poor planning that led to his apprehension, Elton initially described the warehouse as an ideal setup with easy entry and safety because of its proximity to the police station. As the details emerged—the lack of lookouts or an adequate escape plan—Elton shifted and spoke of his real desire to provoke and bait the police, to make them look foolish. "To do that adequately would have required better planning and precautions!" suggested the Doctor. "Look, Doc, I didn't care. I was tired of ripping and running. I needed to get off the streets."

Although the acknowledged game was theft, the significant covert game was to be caught and imprisoned. Elton was tired of the struggle required to maintain himself outside of an institution. Much of his later talk with other men centered on other convicts and prison experiences. As incredible as it seems, Elton could better cope with the rigorous structure of prison than the unstructured street life. Jail, with all of its drawbacks, provided an organization for his life that he was unable to create for himself. It provided food, shelter, a job, clear and identifiable dangers, and a system of guards and procedures upon which he could focus his rage. After all, the system was responsible for his situation and problems!

7. As indicated earlier in the discussion of different treatment approaches, there is a paradox that arises in treatment. Effective treatment must be voluntary. Impulsive people frequently come for treatment involuntarily. The person with a destructive character disorder does not see himself as impaired or needing help. Most frequently, he comes to the helper suffering physical discomfort or under legal or social duress. The duress makes him physically available. Unfortunately, he identifies the helper as society's agent, and since he sees as his only

problem the oppressive society he lives in, he is antagonistic to its agent. Thus, the very factors that make him come for help tend to negate his capacity to accept it. To deal with this, one needs to be pragmatic in terms of what the patient values, not what the helper values.

> Stepan is a 42-year-old plumber with a history of drug abuse and a long standing history of violence. He agreed to an admission to a psychiatric service for an evaluation as an alternative to his wife's pressing charges against him for assault. For several months prior to admission, he had believed that his wife was having an affair. He and his wife had been in counseling as a couple for a considerable time without any significant alterations in their marital relationship. At the time of admission, Stepan was addicted to opiates and showed no signs of psychosis, aside from a generalized suspiciousness. He refused to participate in any of the evaluation meetings and intimidated the staff by flexing his muscles and alluding to past criminal activity.
>
> A senior psychiatrist was called in to help deal with Stepan, who was demanding that he be allowed to sign out of the hospital immediately. Because of his threats toward others and his menacing behavior on the ward, it was clear that he would have to go to another hospital with a locked-door capacity if he should attempt to leave before an evaluation was completed. Stepan knew this, even though he demanded to be allowed to sign out. As the tone of the interview hardened, Stepan made it clear that he could physically destroy the three staff members with whom he was talking. He welcomed the idea of a struggle and began shouting that he wanted to fight with all of the staff at once.
>
> At this point, the senior psychiatrist asked the rest of the staff to leave and sat down to talk to Stepan alone. He acknowledged that there was no comparison between their physical strengths. That was not the issue. Instead, he focused on the likelihood that Stepan would have to spend time in a large hospital and perhaps return to prison, should any of his activities come into the open. "I don't know why you are acting like such an asshole. For a man with your skill in avoiding involvement with the police, it

would seem that you are asking for trouble this time. I can't understand it." Stepan was surprised at the blunt comments and replied, "I don't know, Doc. That is the only way I know how to be. *I ain't never going to change.*"

The psychiatrist then asked how long he had been hopeless about himself. Stepan looked surprised and responded angrily, saying, "That's not what I said." The doctor responded, "You certainly did, you said that you saw no possibility of being anything different, that you'd have to go on making asshole judgments." At that point, Stepan became furious, blew out his breath, and glared at the doctor. The doctor responded, "Well, how else can you look at what you said?" Stepan said nothing. The doctor said, "How long have you been feeling hopeless, and what are you so hopeless about?" Stepan stated sadly that he always felt this way, that other people were smarter, and that the one thing that he valued in life was his family, his children. The doctor then asked why he would jeopardize his relationship with his children by risking hospitalization and imprisonment, all for the minor issue of spending several more days in the hospital. After realizing and discussing the hopelessness he felt with regard to his wife, his children, and himself, Stepan agreed to stay in the hospital. There were no further struggles. The patient valued his freedom and access to his family. The psychiatrist presented his puzzlement as to why the patient would unnecessarily risk losing what he valued.

In this example, as in many that will follow, the patient could not acknowledge that a personal problem existed or that he suffered internal discomfort. This denial represented an attempt to avoid the pervasive and panic-laden sense of hopelessness. Because he felt all attempts at personal change were futile and that he was basically inadequate, he spent a great deal of energy blaming others—society, family, and laws. The drug addict may say, "I've got no problem. It's society that made drugs illegal. Make them legal and I won't have any problem." The criminal says, "I didn't ask to be sent here (jail). I just got caught. That's your problem. You are supposed to rehabilitate me." The alcoholic says, "I just had a little too much. I know I can handle liquor. I've learned my lesson. This won't happen again." The person who has repeatedly attempted suicide frequently says, "I didn't ask to live. The police happened to find me and bring me here. You people saved me. That's your problem." All such statements help the patient to mask his desperation and his own role in creating his problem.

While all of these statements deny the wish for help, skillful therapists can help the patient see that his life experiences are not a series of random incidents designed by fate. Instead, they represent a repetitive, self-created pattern in which he attempts (albeit unsuccessfully) to deal with his own personality problems. Though the patient believes that such thoughtful examination of his behavior is too dangerous and futile, it is my view that the patient's solution, that of avoidance, is the real danger.

In order to overcome the treatment paradox, the helper needs to avoid the traps of diversionary struggles. To do this, he must give to the patient reasons for involvement in treatment that come from the patient's value system, not those of the helper or of society. Thus, the helper may have to see and value the skill required to avoid arrest or the ingenuity involved in a well-conceived confidence game. Questions conceived in this framework help the individual to begin observing and evaluating his own behavior.

It should be apparent to the reader that my strongest bias relates to the possibility of treatment and character change. Clearly stated, most people with destructive character problems (addicts, alcoholics, criminals, borderline personalities, etc.) and many people who have been designated as chronically mentally ill have a far greater potential for growth and alteration than either they or their therapists believe. The process is arduous, painful, and time-consuming. It involves numerous setbacks. The process of change, however, is ultimately less painful than a lifetime of chronic, desperate, destructive activity.

CHAPTER 2

The Settings and the People

Lexington

My most concentrated clinical experience with impulsive individuals occurred during 2 years spent in the U.S. Public Health Service. This time was spent at the National Institute of Mental Health, Clinical Research Center, Lexington, Kentucky, also known as the "Narcotics Farm" or NARCO.

Within this setting, I had significant contact with approximately 1,000 male[1] opiate addicts and polydrug abusers and intensive contact with approximately 400. These 400 men were seen in conferences, in group and individual therapy sessions. Unless otherwise indicated, the case histories throughout the book stem from my Lexington experience.

The hospital is set on 900 acres of rolling countryside in Lexington, Kentucky. Architecturally, the buildings resemble a

[1] Although the book contains clinical examples of men and women patients, the text is written in terms of the patients as men. In part, this is a response to the fact that the author's experiences are primarily with male patients. It also is easier in terms of writing to speak in terms of a single gender. Many of the issues are applicable to both men and women. Some issues apply more to one sex. Because the book is intended as a presentation of general issues for beginners in the field, I have not attempted to distinguish the specific issues of men or women who are impulsive.

prison, with narrow steel windows and completely enclosed courtyards. Until 1968, the institution was managed as a prison. Steel fences surrounded the entire complex and barbed wire topped the walls. Doorways were bounded by prison grills and bars. Guards kept the "patients" moving in the hallways, to the extent that the men had to face the walls when women went by.

One former guard reported that he felt he was supposed to shout at the patients all day: "Keep moving. No talking. No loitering." He began disliking himself and his job. Soon, this bitterness focused upon the patients, whom he came to resent for causing him to participate in a dehumanizing process.

Minimal provocations caused some guards to exercise their power and put patients in the "hole." At the same time, there were many humane staff members who tried on an individual basis to assist patients. However, there was no training for staff or group commitment to the rehabilitation program by staff and patients. The pessimism inherent in the addict was supported by the dehumanizing process. His basic style of blaming others for his status was reinforced by the reality of the treatment and rehabilitation program.

In 1968, many elements of the prisonlike atmosphere—the bars, the barbed wire, and the hole—were removed, and the guards were no longer allowed free access to the treatment units. The enunciated policy was to view addicts as human beings. But, this well-intentioned and necessary first step was not followed by the delineation of a program for training, treatment, and research. What ensued was a short period of freedom from responsibility and obligation that resulted in chaos within the institution. The staff and the patients lost their defined roles and became more depressed.

A new director was appointed at this time. Because of the preexisting situation and personality conflicts he became a focus of anger. In spite of this, he furthered the development of a treatment program. He enunciated the policy of greater freedom for the patients based upon the demonstration of responsible behavior. He also asked the unit chiefs and the staff of the five treatment subunits to develop their own style of treatment.

Previously, the unit chiefs had been physicians and psychiatrists who were fulfilling their 2-year government service. Thus, every 2 years, there had to be a traumatic reorganization as one group of professionals left and a new group of professionals entered the institution as unit directors. The new director appointed career Public Health Service nurses, social workers, and psychologists to become permanent unit chiefs. This helped to stabilize the treatment units and gave them a sense of permanence. The middle-echelon clinical staff, composed of physicians fulfilling their service commitment, still changed every 2 years. By 1970, the units began to make more realistic performance demands of the patients. The period of complete freedom ended, without a return to the old system of a punitive prison setting.

The unit in which I worked opened in May of 1970. Previously, it had been the centralized withdrawal and detoxification unit for the whole hospital. Staff members had worked well with each other and felt comfortable in their medical roles. The unit chief was a male nurse who had come to the hospital in 1969; the head nurse, a woman, served as staff spokesperson. In July of 1970, I joined the unit staff. The unit chief, the head nurse, another physician, and myself formed a nuclear group that shared the belief that effective change in the patients could come through active staff participation in a defined treatment program.

Many of the staff members had years of government service and training that had instilled in them the desire merely to take orders. Although they complained about the ineptitude of their superiors, they were hesitant to participate openly in the process of treatment design and review. They did not see that carrying out orders in an unenthusiastic, possibly hostile manner would communicate a lack of personal conviction destructive to treatment. The already skeptical patients viewed the world as a place in which there are only those who give orders and those who take orders. To further substantiate this belief in the individual's powerlessness to affect his situation by providing a passive compliant staff would be disastrous. Many staff members seemed to have become relatively comfortable in their passive, complaining roles: "I'm only an aide"; "I'm only a GS-3, I'm not supposed to talk about that."

As a counter measure to this entrenched passivity, all staff members were given an equal role in making policy decisions. Each staff member was given a single vote on policy decisions. A veto power was retained by the unit director but was never needed. Thus, the unit director and the nurses' aide had an equal say in policy decisions. In fact, because there were more nurses and aides, they could easily outvote the unit director. The decision to function in this manner incorporated a conscious decision to risk mistakes and disagreement in order to form a more cohesive and positively involved staff.

At first, the majority of the staff continued in their passive roles. When it was pointed out that the staff continued to use the same weak excuses as the addicts to explain their lack of involvement, they reacted by voting down every administrative proposal for the next 3 months. As these issues were repeatedly confronted and argued in the staff meetings, the tone of the unit changed. People came in on days off to attend staff meetings (unheard of in government service).

Another significant change arose from the nuclear group's belief that the patients should have the right to question the staff about their behavior within the institution. Initially, this meant that the nurses and aides were asked to *participate* as leaders in group therapy sessions and to relinquish their silent, observer roles.

The staff was extremely uncomfortable with the proposal to allow patients to observe staff activities and question members. Their previously defined role was no longer secure. The patients tended to pressure the overtly uncomfortable staff members, thus increasing their distress.

As a support to the staff, demonstration interviews and teaching conferences were repeated several times a week. One day, staff tension was particularly noticeable on the unit. When asked to discuss with the staff the source of their discomfort, I was criticized for making the staff feel inadequate and demanding too much. As we discussed these issues, it became apparent that in many instances I had been wrong.

Temporary relief followed, along with a decision to hold such meetings weekly. It was becoming clear that administrators and physicians—those nominally in charge—could be questioned and criticized. No longer did staff members need to feel like powerless robots who resentfully carried out orders.

Not all of the staff could tolerate these changes, which seemed to negate much of their personal life experiences. Some staff members transferred from the unit to other units in the center. Many who remained on the unit, as well as those who transferred in, experienced a sense of excitement about their work. As they and others began to value their active participation, their self-esteem rose.

Open staff meetings with the patients became the major issue. Most staff members were still afraid that these would leave them vulnerable to manipulation and dissatisfaction on the part of the patients. Some feared the loss of intimate private relationships with patients that served as a source of information and pride. The nuclear group, on the other hand, felt that such "secret" information was useless and destructive since it eliminated the patients' participation in the group. A goal of the open meetings was to promote the understanding and confidence of the patients, who previously had believed that the staff would secretly decide all issues regardless of patient thoughts, behavior, or needs.

With great resistance, all meetings except one were opened to participation by patients. The result was a noticeable lessening of complaints about the staff and its way of operating. As the men saw the process of discussion, disagreement, resolution, and planning, they began to understand its validity for their own work.

For a considerable period of time, the tendency to passivity within the staff was evidenced in the lack of creative suggestions from the nurses, aides, and social workers. Later, with increasing self-esteem, they began to regroup, suggest changes, and organize innovative alterations within the program. They even began to risk the possibility of openly making mistakes and reviewing them.

The patients, by and large, still did not share the goals of the staff but did adopt from them certain role model positions. The patients became more involved than ever before.

One of the difficulties that had not been overcome was the time limitation imposed by the courts on a person's stay in the program. Because of the maximum 6 months, there was a constant turnover of patients. This had a disruptive effect and impeded progress. Therapy groups rarely coalesced, and the limited goal of the staff became that of sensitizing the individual to seeing his own role in creating the situations in which he became embroiled. This meant getting him to stop seeing others as responsible for his trouble and to begin examining the basis of his own behavior.

With each improvement in the functioning of the unit, there developed a strong tendency to accept the new improvement as sufficient. Each time there was a positive change (patients working, going to school, and participating in therapy and in the program), the staff felt a sense of satisfaction and a fear of returning to the turmoil that was always necessary to make further changes and gains.

Both patients and staff verbally acknowledged that there was a long way to go. But each time increasing demands were placed upon them, conflict ensued. *There was an inherent danger in the program of seeing each new level of achievement as an end from which there was no need for further growth.*

In order for growth to occur, turmoil is necessary. People must struggle together to iron out differences and develop means of change. They must openly deal with reservations, hopes, and fears. A calm and stable situation within a hospital or a treatment setting may indicate only a new level of comfortable chronicity. *Turmoil is a constant and necessary ingredient for growth, and growth is the purpose of social institutions.*

The colleague mentioned in the Introduction, who found that it was the staff's aim to fill its wards with quiet patients, encountered major resistance when he fought to change the system. His staff resented the intrusion of acutely disorganized patients who upset the routine and agitated the other, more quiet individuals. As he began instituting treatment beyond chronic care, staff anxiety rose sharply. Because his staff members did not understand such treatment as possible for their patients or as something they could usefully participate in, some resisted the change, and others ventilated their disagreement. Only by working through these disagreements could they attain a system allowing increased patient care. After 2 years, his staff members were enthusiastically involved in patient care and resented any implication that they were working in a *chronic* (hopeless) hospital.

The Composite Patient at Lexington

The composite man at Lexington during 1970–1972 was 23 years old with a 10th-grade education. By age 15, 33% of the men were seriously abusing alcohol. By age 18, 41% were using nonopiate drugs. By 19, the average man in this group was regularly using opiate drugs. At the time of his admission, the period of consistent abuse was 3.5 years.

The economic background can best be described as poor to lower-middle-class. There were some professionals and some persons from wealthy families, but they accounted for less than 5% of the population at the hospital.

Of the patients, 50% had physically healthy mothers in their homes until age 18. An additional 15% had alcoholic mothers, 5% had mothers addicted to opiates, and 5% had mothers who were opiate-dependent during the course of a prolonged terminal illness. In general, the mothers of these men tended to fall into two categories: overly indulgent women and women who were disinterested in their children's growth and development.

Upon close examination, the overindulgence shown by

many mothers was actually disinterest or hostility. It frequently represented the way in which the mother could put out the least effort in the care of the child. These mothers would not set adequate limits for attendance at school or demand appropriate behavior of their children when they were caught in delinquent acts. Some mothers repeatedly uttered disbelief each time their children got into serious difficulties with the law. Many of these mothers, while asking the young addict to give up his addiction, supplied money that went to support the habit, and in some cases, the mothers actually purchased the drug when the addict was too sick to obtain it for himself. These inconsistencies between expressed maternal interest and actual maternal behavior appear to be germaine in the design of treatment. Similar contradictory behavior in treatment settings promotes a reawakening of the initial despair and hopelessness. This early interaction necessitates the treatment staff to be both *reasonable and consistent in words and actions.* Inconsistency reduplicates the early developmental experiences. Giving in to excessive and unreasonable demands as his mother did becomes a disruptive experience to the patient. He wants reasonable reactions and a new parent.

Other mothers were described as cold, distant, depressed, or disinterested. These women were emotionally unavailable to their children, either because they were preoccupied with maintaining the household or because they were so withdrawn into their own emotional issues that they could not care for their children.

A number of these mothers appeared to be acting out their hostility toward men through their male offspring. In response to this, a significant number of the men classified themselves as "mama's boys" until early adolescence. At that point, the typical patient reacted to the conflicting demands and behavior of his mother by behaving in a manner that was designed to provoke her into being available and consistent. This frequently involved behaving like the previously disparaged father or father substitute.

In a sense, the emphasis upon the mother's role may be skewed. However pathologic the relationship, she tended to be present and available for some kind of interaction. Fathers represented a much more unstable group. They were frequently absent or only occasionally physically present. Emotionally, they tended to be unavailable to their wives and children. They were, when present, impulsive, alcoholic, abusive, inconsistent, remote, overcontrolling, or passive. Only 26% of the men had fathers available to them up to age 18 who were not severely emotionally disabled. Another 15% had severely alcoholic fathers in the home until age 18. The rest (59%) had fathers or father substitutes in the home only intermittently until age 18. When available in the home, 50% of all the fathers were physically abusive men who took no constructive role in raising their children. How much is the lack of a father figure a factor in the ongoing process of struggling with society's authorities (police, courts, etc.)? *Is this struggle really the struggle of children to deal with the inconsistent and intermittently present father?* Does the impulse-ridden person force society to provide the stern controlling father of early childhood?

Racially, the patients at Lexington were approximately 60% black and 40% white. Whether this represents an adequate reflection of the distribution of drug use in the general population or is a function of the process of selection by society is not clear.[2] Entry into Lexington usually meant that community resources for the treatment of drug addiction had been exhausted. Prior to their admission to the hospital at Lexington, 75% of the men had spent time in jail. Only 10% had never been arrested. And 60% of the men entered the program by agreement with prosecutors or judges that the treatment program would act as an alternative to serving prison terms or facing prosecution for drug-related crimes. The men's previous criminal experience ran the gamut from murder, rape, and assault to forgery and petty larceny. Those who entered the hospital without formal legal pressure

[2] My Lexington unit served the southern United States.

frequently did so in response to family pressure or as a means of avoiding potential prosecution in their home districts.

In general, the men who entered this unit had exhausted treatment means in their own communities or had come from communities that had none available. They had quit or had been thrown out of self-help units. They used methadone in combination with other drugs or sold methadone for other opiates. Some had been drug counselors and group leaders in communities while they used drugs. Thus, the men in this study represented the "street addict," everybody's treatment failure. Upon admission, the addict was not interested in rehabilitation. *How can there be rehabilitation from a prolonged life experience in which drugs are only one of a long series of self-destructive acts?* If his condition prior to drug use was never satisfactory, the concept of *re*habilitation was senseless, and this deception was apparent to the patient: he had never been "habilitated" to begin with. He saw the institution as another way of "doing time" jailhouse style. The fact that doors were open, that there were no guards or bars, that he had his own room and enjoyed a modified self-government did not affect his attitudes or beliefs. To him, it was just another jail.

The patients entered with the following three basic beliefs:

1. "Everyone—the staff, the doctors, and the patients—is a con man. They may do it in a different way, but, in fact, they are no different from me. If they are deceptive and dishonest, why should I change? There is really no difference, except for the way the con is done, the style."

2. "I can get anything, if I just learn how to work it. So I gotta learn more angles for working things." (This we later discuss as *manipulation*.)

3. "People who get uptight at lies and deceit are really phony. Everyone is a con man. They're just fooling themselves. In fact, I am more honest than those hypocrites. I don't hide what I am. If you're not a deceptive con man, you're a sucker. Those are the only two choices in life, con man or sucker, on top or on bottom."

A Psychiatric Hospital Setting

A number of examples are drawn from my experience as a psychiatrist working with hospitalized psychiatric patients. Here the setting was a community of 250,000 people in the northeastern United States. Although surrounded by wealthy suburbs, the community was basically poor, made up of many closely knit ethnic and racial minority groups. The psychiatric unit was a 30-bed voluntary unit located in an old building adjacent to the main medical facility.

The staff—both professional and nonprofessional—were young and energetic. The psychiatric service was new to the hospital and attracted many young and dedicated individuals whose goal was the development of community-oriented psychiatric service.

Initially, staff members at the inpatient service had viewed themselves and their work as an extension of their commitment to changing United States society. Young, idealistic, and energetic, they had not developed the cynicism initially present in the staff at Lexington. Believing in the inherent goodness of men and their own goodwill, they enthusiastically jumped into the process of treatment. The senior staff provided training and supervision, yet there was a resistance to the more traditional and organized approaches to patient evaluation and care. An outgrowth of the idealism of the mid 1960s and the disappointment of the early 1970s was an antagonism to older, more established approaches to patients and learning. The concept of setting limits and expectations seemed potentially repressive. Issues, such as evaluating behavior for consistency prior to sanctioning time off the ward, appeared to be a violation of civil rights. Sharing information among the staff members was a compromise of privileged communication. How could there be trust? Requiring attendance at therapy was a limitation of free choice.

These issues became most problematic with the impulse-ridden, self-destructive, but nonpsychotic patients. Verbally skilled and aware of the current social–political rhetoric, these patients taxed the staff's belief in the ultimate goodness of the individual, who needed only to be given more understanding and consideration.

Over a period of months, using the same procedure of staff meetings, discussions, and program planning as described for Lexington, the staff developed a more balanced perspective that included both reasonable structure and appropriate consideration of the rights and dignity of the individual. Interestingly, many of the staff members gave up the idealized beliefs in radically new approaches to treatment that would be quicker and less rigorous. At the same time, they reviewed their own previously discarded interest in formal graduate training. Clearly, their wish to avoid older forms of training was carried into the arena of work. Many have developed an amalgam of traditional training tempered with enthusiasm and experience that seems to lead to a more gradual process of change.

Over a 3-year period, 1972–1975, the number of people seen in the center for impulsive and self-destructive behavior accounted for approximately 30% of the psychiatric admissions. The number might have been larger but for three factors: (1) patients seen primarily as having problems relating to drug or alcohol abuse were usually treated on units designated for alcohol and drug abuse; (2) the emergency-room psychiatric staff became highly skilled at supporting and maintaining impulsively destructive people outside of the hospital; and finally, (3) many wildly out-of-control individuals were sent to the involuntary state hospital until they reorganized.

In spite of these factors, 30% of the more than 300 yearly admissions were people like Stepan (p. 20). As was the case at Lexington, the majority of these people came from homes where one parent was transient; and alcoholism, physical abuse, and economic privation occurred. There were a substantial number of individuals who had grown up in economically secure homes with both parents physically present. In these settings, parental inconsistency and lack of realistic demands and limits were frequently coupled with alcoholism and emotional unavailability.

Most of the patients with impulsive and destructive behavior were young people ranging from 18 to 35 years old. It was unusual to find someone over 35 years of age who acted in this manner.

An Outpatient Clinic for Drug Abusers

In 1972, I began weekly consultations to an outpatient clinic set up to work with male heroin and polydrug addicts. Most of the young men had served in Vietnam and received some veterans' benefits. Many of these individuals attributed their drug abuse to the Vietnam experience. However, factual clinical histories revealed drug and alcohol abuse as well as impulsive behavior prior to entry into the service. Some of these men had entered the armed forces as a way of having criminal charges dropped. Many others looked to the service to add structure and organization to their lives (parental functions).

One of the primary functions of the clinic was methadone dispensing for maintenance and detoxification. In addition, group and individual therapy as well as job counseling were available. The clinic was located in an old building in the business section of a large eastern city. This was convenient to transportation for the men, who came from many sections of the metropolitan area.

Unlike Lexington and the psychiatric inpatient unit, the clinic had no overnight facility or day-care responsibilities for its patients. These men came daily or several times a week for various combinations of therapy and/or methadone. In 1972, the clinic was still new, and I found the staff struggling with the same problems that the other two units I had worked in had faced. What were reasonable expectations, and what was punitive? What constituted compromises of civil rights and confidentiality? What were the responsibilities of the staff to the patients? What were the patient's responsibilities? How does one deal with the impulsive behavior occurring outside of the clinic? What can I do? Can anything be done? It became apparent that no matter what the setting or the patient designation, staff and patients would ultimately have to deal with similar basic issues.

CHAPTER 3

Character Disorders

Some form of destructive personality disorder is characteristic of many addicts. It will be useful to take a closer look at these disorders.

It is difficult for the layman to understand a destructive personality disorder. A person with this kind of problem does not complain of his symptoms or seek help for them as does the neurotic, nor does he show the confusion of the psychotic. He can speak rationally and persuasively. Because his destructive, impulsive, and irresponsible behavior is carried out consciously and deliberately, one cannot attribute it to a deranged mental process.

Character develops as a result of the interaction of the individual's constitution with the environment. This usually begins with the mother, then the other family members, and gradually an expanding number of individuals and institutions within the community. If, as one grows, adequate affection is lacking, if parents and adult models fall short, and if inconsistent, untrustworthy, violent, and destructive models take their place, then these become the individual's norms. Thus, the person with such a character disorder does not see antisocial, delinquent, destructive behavior as abnormal. For him, it's just his way of getting along.

Destructive personality in this sense frequently leads us to think of economic deprivation, ghettos, etc. In such settings one comes to expect more open and harsh struggles for existence and a more apparent desperation. But the same lack of structure, limits, positive goals, affection, satisfaction, and consistent parental relationships can be found in middle-class and wealthy suburbs. The well-cared-for home also contains alcoholism, indifference, preoccupied parents, and the substitution of material goods for affection. A person who grows up with a sense of emptiness and inadequacy will develop a need for immediate gratification and will be unable to tolerate discomfort and frustration.

These needs are the norm for the person with destructive personality. He has never felt any different. He does not discern one part of himself that is uncomfortable as contrasted with areas of success and self-respect. To acknowledge that he has a problem would be devastating, because it leads to an awareness that others do not have the same constant and generalized distress. From this, he must conclude that there are other, more comfortable ways of being that he has not experienced and fears he may never be able to experience. As one man stated after reviewing his history and seeing this perspective, "My God, Doc, if what we're talking about is true, that's my whole life, that's me! There's *nothing* there!" Subsequently, he gave up the "if" in his statement and experienced a massive depression from which he had been running for many years.

The street addict usually falls into one of the following subcategories listed in the *Diagnostic and Statistical Manual of the American Psychiatric Association* (DSM-2) and somewhat simplified here. *These categories of personality disorders are listed to demonstrate the clinical uselessness and sterility of using such descriptions for anything more than categorizing.* They tell us little that is helpful in our work.

Personality Disorders

Paranoid

This behavior is characterized by hypersensitivity, rigidity, unwarranted suspicion, jealousy, envy, excessive self-importance, and a tendency to blame others and ascribe evil motives to them.

Schizoid

A person with this behavior pattern manifests shyness and oversensitivity. He avoids close or competitive relationships. Apparently, he lives in fantasy but without loss of capacity to recognize reality. Daydreaming is common, and he may be unable to express hostility and ordinary aggressive feelings. These patients react to disturbing experiences and conflicts with apparent detachment.

Explosive

This behavior is characterized by gross outbursts of rage or of verbal or physical aggressiveness. These outbursts are strikingly different from the patient's usual behavior, and he may regret them. These patients are generally considered excitable, aggressive, and overresponsive to environmental pressures. It is the intensity of the outbursts and the inability to control them that distinguishes this group. Patients we diagnose as "aggressive personality" fall in this group.

Antisocial

This term is reserved for persons whose behavior brings them repeatedly into conflict with society. They are incapable of significant loyalty to individuals, groups, or social values. They are grossly selfish, callous, irresponsible, impulsive, and unable to feel guilt or to learn from experience and punishment. Frustration tolerance is low. They tend to blame others or to offer plausible rationalizations for their behavior. A mere history of repeated legal or social offenses is not sufficient to justify this diagnosis.

Passive-Aggressive

This behavior is characterized by both passivity and aggressiveness. The patient may express aggressiveness passively, by being obstructive, intentionally inefficient, or stubborn. This behavior commonly reflects hostility that the patient does not dare express openly. Often it is an expression of resentment at failing to find gratification in a relationship with an individual or an institution upon which he is overdependent.

Borderline Personalities [1]

An individual with a borderline personality forms an immediate and intense relationship characterized by great expectations or a harsh rejection of the individual with whom he is forming the relationship. He has the capacity for showing immediate and severe regressions evidenced by destructive behavior (alcoholic binges, wrist cutting, overdosing, or brief periods of frank psychosis). The psychosis itself is usually outgoing in nature, not involving withdrawal. The person will involve many people in rescuing him at this point. Such an individual has intense needs and demands that, when unmet, cause him to fly into a self-destructive rage. He is labile, given to sharp mood swings. Frequently, such a person functions in a bisexual manner.

Depression

Having become acquainted with these general diagnostic labels, one may now more usefully view these personalities in terms of manifest behavior and try to understand their dynamic origins. A sense of the patient's pervasive emptiness, depression, and panic emerges. Examples follow the behavioral descriptions.

Low Self-Esteem

Patients with destructive personalities usually evidence little that they value about themselves. Many show excessive bravado, especially in the presence of people whom they view as different or better off than themselves. This is seen as an over-

---

[1] Not mentioned in DSM-2 but a generally accepted diagnostic entity.

compensation for their discomfort with people who do not share their propensity for self-destruction. Even among themselves, however, any minor slight, intentional or accidental, becomes cause for serious confrontation. Their fragile sense of self-esteem is always hanging in the balance. Behind it is the question, "Am I really a valuable person?" Because of this nagging self-doubt, there are constant efforts to substantiate the external image without resolving the internal doubts. Thus, an individual will risk physical danger or imprisonment at the slightest provocation, in order to maintain his self-esteem.

> Bill, a short man, was leaning against a Ping-Pong table. He was asked to move by Wendell, an extremely tall, muscular individual. Bill, sensitive about his size, thought he detected an insult in Wendell's voice. While Bill knew he was in the way, he refused to move and challenged Wendell to move him. The two were stopped just short of a fight. At a minimum, both risked leaving the hospital and returning to prison; at a maximum, death, for each acknowledged that he had been prepared to kill the other. Bill later explained in group, "I'm nothing, but it would kill me to let those suckers know it. I've gotta show them all the time. It would just kill me if they knew. Then I'd really be nothing."

Many such life-and-death struggles have developed over a book of matches, a place in line, or a game of pool. Such an individual, when seen alone, refers to himself as "a failure" and speaks in anger about things he has not received. This usually leads to a feeling that he lacks some internal strength or capacity, that something is missing. When institutionalized, he makes unrealistic demands for irrational luxuries. Roughly translated, he is saying, "I have been deprived, you have not. Therefore, it is up to you to give to me."

Inability to Form Close Personal Relationships

Addicts tend to change relationships constantly. At Lexington, almost half the men were divorced, and three-quarters described themselves as never having been close to anyone.

In spite of numerous involvements with people, Jim stated it this way, "It's funny, even with a buddy where I know I should feel something, like sympathy or understanding, you know, I feel nothing. I just kinda go through the motions."

Irv, who was superficially engaging, articulate, and poised, described his avoidance of serious personal involvement this way, "Like a man's a really good pimp, until he falls for one of his whores, if he cares, he's finished." This was in keeping with his saying, "Your worst enemy is having a friend." "You're safe if you don't care. Stay cool."

In the predatory world of these men, there are those who are on top and those who are on the bottom. Being on top requires having no allegiance that could drag you down. They see no alternative. This pattern of behavior begins long before the initial use of drugs. In many instances, one is able to trace the avoidance of personal relationships back to early life with parents and family. When an individual loses hope about himself, he gives up on human relationships to avoid and defend against further disappointment and hurt.

Many addicts avoid significant relationships because they perceive themselves as internally weak and inadequate. The addict fears that he will lose his identity by merging or blending with the other person's "stronger" character. This wish for fusion coupled with fear of it emerges in descriptions of the drug experience. It is "safer" with a drug because he feels that he can control it; it is not like losing oneself in another person.

At the same time, he is constantly moving about, changing relationships and seeking a person or a group that will give him a sense of well-being. Because he has failed to resolve his internal conflict between the fear of closeness and the desire for a nonthreatening, all-giving relationship, he is in constant turmoil. This search is partially resolved in the drug experience. While on the drug, he is in a trouble-free state of mind, in which the existence of personal turmoil is transiently diminished.

These fears are constantly demonstrated in the addict's demand that the would-be helper or friend prove his sincerity.

Because no amount of proof will resolve the addict's doubt about his own value and the capacity of others to value him, he constantly tests any relationship in a futile, destructive manner. The hope is to find someone who will resolve the personal doubts and give the individual a sense of self worth that he has not been able to achieve on his own. Unfortunately, there can never be enough external support when such massive internal doubts are unresolved. The would-be counselor can become involved in a perpetual series of tests of his own willingness to give, unless he defines the limits of the relatonship in concrete terms. Doing so helps to eliminate the later disappointment of the addict's unrealistic expectations. The message the therapist needs to convey is:

> "I genuinely care for you, but in a finite way. *I am not all-giving and I do not apologize for that.* All human relationships have limits as to what one person can do for another. Within my personal limits, I shall try to be of assistance to you. I can best assist you by aiding you in doing for yourself. Doing things for you is a disservice as it implies that you cannot do them for yourself."

In practice, this means defining meeting times, goals, areas in which the counselor is of potential use, and areas in which he will not get involved. The patient and counselor also need to understand the consequences of failures to maintain their treatment agreement. As part of the process of defining a treatment agreement, it is important for the patient to clarify what he is going to contribute to the working relationship.

Many counselors who do not define the motives and goals of treatment become involved in running to courts, judges, social workers, and clinics in a perpetual round of efforts to stop the maladaptive and self-destructive behavior or to protect the addict from the consequences of his behavior. The failure to define initial goals only supports the addict's wish and expectation of finding the perfect all-giving person. It is not uncommon to see the addict calmly sitting in his cell or in the judge's chambers while his family or counselor frantically tries to secure his release or ease his sentence. Clearly, the roles have been reversed. It is the addict who should be expending the effort, demonstrating his desire to help himself by his behavior, not the alleged helper.

Manipulation

This word refers to the use of deceit, distortion, misrepresentation, and of all the other methods that the person uses to get others to do something for him. To most people, this term conjures up a critical sense of condemnation. To the impulse-ridden person, it is the skill upon which he bases his hope of success. It is the major tool of his life's trade. He prides himself on his ability to use and improve his skill of "conning."

> Sam is a 30-year-old with several years of college education. He sought individual therapy ostensibly because "I want to change, to stop doing all this shit." With a superficially depressed attitude, he recalled his early childhood of deprivation. Later, he listed numbers of doctors whom he had deceived into giving him drugs. His voice conveyed no genuine emotional involvement, nor was there any evidence of serious desire to alter himself in the current situation. He was asked, "Since we both know you like to con people, especially doctors, I wonder if you are doing this with me now and how it would help you?" He became visibly uncomfortable and later revealed that his visits with the therapist helped him avoid involvement in his group therapy. Any issue directed to him he deferred from the group therapy to the individual session: "I'm talking that over with the psychiatrist." In neither setting would he focus upon himself and his own sense of failing.

Behind the dependence upon manipulation is a message: *"I have no confidence in my own ability to accomplish tasks or achieve goals for myself. If I let people know what I want, they will certainly deny it to me. I must therefore deceive people and use them to get for me what I cannot get for myself.* Manipulation is the patient's acknowledgment of his own emotional bankruptcy.

Many therapists become angry when they find that they have been manipulated. This anger may represent an injury to the therapist's pride (narcissism) in that he felt that the patient would not or could not manipulate him. In part, this is because the therapist feels intellectually superior to the addict and has been proven wrong. In part, he feels that he has some skills and interests that other people don't have and that therefore the addict should treat and value him differently than others. The bias may represent the therapist's belief that in fact he is better than the patient in an existential or a qualitative way. These are human responses that the therapist must be alert to if he is to learn about himself in order to be useful to his patient. If he only reacts to the provocation and fails to understand his own response, he forecloses the option of exploring the patient's particular need for deception and provocation. The chance for both to learn about the patient's choice of this mode of interaction is then lost. It is appropriate for the therapist to be alert for manipulative traps and to attempt to avoid them. His approach needs to be open and frank. When he finds that he has fallen into a manipulation, he needs to acknowledge it and explore with the patient what purpose it has served. He must constantly push the patient to see the defensive nature of the manipulation and then focus on the issue that the patient could not face. What did the manipulation help him to avoid?

In order to do this, the therapist needs to be aware of his own limitations and to be comfortable with himself as a fallible person. If he becomes angered at a manipulation, he falls into a second trap. His anger supports the addict's basic belief that all people are con men and that he and the therapist are involved in a game of one-upmanship. He correctly perceives that the therapist's anger has resulted from the therapist's disappointment at having been "one-upped" by the patient.

The above does not mean that a therapist must be an excessively lenient or accepting person. Once the limits, goals, expectations, and consequences have been agreed upon by therapist and patient, they must be adhered to firmly. These patients need and find it useful to have a therapist who is practical, realistic, and dependable.

Barbara is a 28-year-old divorced model with a history of prostitution, drug addiction, alcoholism, multiple suicide attempts, and assaultive behavior. She was admitted to an open psychiatric ward of a general hospital during a period of serious depression. She had been admitted with the understanding that she would have no visitors or use of drugs. It was a clear expectation upon admission that she would discuss her impulses rather than act upon them and would avoid any sexual involvement with patients or staff. She was expected to use good judgment at all times. Two days after admission, she was found in bed with another patient. She had been bored and had sought the involvement for transient relief. She had arranged the sexual liaison openly; it was clearly an invitation to be caught. She had stated that she could not tolerate the hospital and was seeking a way of getting thrown out. Further discussion in her group led to a reemergence of the hopeless feeling that she had been avoiding and an angry criticism of the hospital for not making her less depressed immediately. The patient was not psychotic and had clearly decided on her course of action. When this was put in the context of her admission agreement, it was decided that she could not stay, and she was sent to another hospital because of increasing suicidal preoccupations. The other hospital was a large, understaffed custodial institution that did not provide the comforts of the more adequately arranged general hospital.

Barbara called 2 days after admission to the other hospital to say that she had dramatically improved, was less depressed, and wanted to return to the general hospital to work on the chronic issues of her impulsive behavior and recurrent depressions. She was readmitted with an agreement similar to that of her previous admission. She became a model patient, active in therapy groups and in individual therapy sessions. Then, 1 week after the second admission, she revealed that she had been using drugs on the previous night. The group and the therapist were so moved by her ability to share herself openly that they decided to forego the initial treatment agreement with regard to drug use. The patient was transiently elated upon hearing this and talked about the warm feelings that she had had when she realized their understanding of her.

Several hours later, she made a serious suicide attempt; she remained severely depressed with a surge of suicidal intentions. The staff increased their commitment to help her through this difficult time, but *the patient deteriorated as the staff's efforts increased.* After a tumultuous period, that finally required electric shock treatment to reduce the suicidal pressure, the patient returned to the custodial hospital and was discharged 1 week later. She resumed treatment as an outpatient at the general hospital.

Reconstruction of these episodes revealed that her punitive conscience, which had failed to get the group to punish her for her behavior (drug use), could not tolerate the positive caring response to her. She felt so unworthy that she had to punish herself. Her conscience then inflicted upon her a serious punishing depression unlike any other that she had experienced in the past. Medication and human interaction failed to alter it. People's caring efforts only enhanced her need for punishment. She was unworthy. Electroshock, in a sense a punishment, temporarily relieved the pressure she experienced. Failure to abide by the agreement that both parties had worked out before her second admission led to this need for extreme self-punishment. Had there been a different agreement or a negotiated alteration in the agreement, some of the anguish and removal to a state hospital might have been avoided. Agreements need to be adhered to or reasonably altered through mutual resolution.

Clearly, none of us wishes to see himself as inflicting punishment upon his patients. Nor does one wish to satisfy the patient's desire for punishment. Many addicts and criminals give histories that indicate that they have set themselves up repeatedly for punishment and arrest. As unbelievable as it may seem to the new worker, *many of these individuals whose behavior is so reprehensible live with a severely punishing conscience that seeks out punishment by individuals and society.* Unfortunately, they get involved in a cyclical system of criminal activity leading to punishment. The punishment inflicted by others leads to a transient sense of relief, which becomes freedom to commit more crimes and seek further punishment.

It is the therapist's job, however, to explore the basis for the patient's behavior. He must neither rescue the patient nor morally judge him. His only job is to help the patient to see his personal role in creating his difficulties, to understand the motivation for this behavior, and to try to find satisfying ways of resolving these inner conflicts.

When focusing upon the need for manipulation, the therapist usually discovers the hopelessness and emptiness that developed early in the patient's life. Manipulation has its origin in beliefs that one is helpless, hopeless, and worthless.

Nonpsychotic Techniques of Avoidance

Projection, displacement, denial, and distortion are nonpsychotic techniques of avoidance. They are an attempt to place the focus of the problem outside of oneself. The addict uses them to explain his personal failure in terms of the social system, family, government, schools, race, or religion. These statements usually boil down to the following: "If X had been different in my life, then I would not have turned out this way. Because I cannot change the past, I cannot be any different."

A sense of mourning and anger over some early deprivation pervades these harangues. However, when he mentions his early losses, the addict is frequently not interested in exploring the truth that may, in part, underlie his statements. Many times his only interest is in establishing a cause-and-effect relationship that absolves him of responsibility or shares the blame with others. Frequently, he becomes expert at pointing out the genuine and significant failures in his environment. He does not, however, deal with the issue that his use of drugs in no way rectifies the environmental failures. He seeks only an excuse for his continued self-destruction, not a constructive explanation leading to positive change. He relishes the news reports of high officials caught in illicit activities and delights in the therapist's discomfort as the therapist reluctantly acknowledges the use of alcohol or marijuana. He fails to discern the difference between the functioning staff member with many areas of success who has occasionally used drugs and his own situation of chronic failure. It is the role of the staff to clarify this inconsistent logic and face the addict with the reality of the situation *without moralizing*. The task is to help him explore the origin and development of his pattern of behavior.

> Calvin was explaining an impulsive series of actions that had led him into conflict with various institutions. After some discussion, he said, "I don't know why I do these things. I just do them. I feel like it. I don't know why!" When pressed further to explain the repetitious quality of his behavior, he became angry at the therapist, criticizing his approach. The therapist refused to discuss his approach, nor the attempt to sidetrack the discussion into an angry interchange. Calvin had tried to shift the focus of attention to the therapist's style. He further projected his anger when he began impugning the therapist's motivation for his questions. He angrily accused the therapist of being critical and punitive: "You think you're different! Better than me!" Both were projections of his own demeaned self, which constantly devalued him. The questions about his behavior persisted. He became visibly upset and responded, "I don't like to think about those things [the clear repetitive behavior pattern]. They make me depressed. Once I get depressed, I don't think I will ever get better." Calvin avoided depression as if once he experienced it he would never feel better again. He was showing the basic lack of a sense of well-being that allows one to tolerate mood shifts into depression and sadness. Most of us can buoy ourselves through depressive episodes by noting other areas of self-respect and remembering that we have successfully been through bad times before.

Inability to Examine One's Own Behavior

Several defenses to avoid self-evaluation have been discussed. Left to his own devices, the addict will continue to act self-destructively. When shown the part he played in reaching his current status, he becomes noticeably uncomfortable. The sense of personal failure, emptiness, and impotence from which he has been running begins to emerge.

Previously, he has used drugs or activity to ignore these feelings. Within the treatment setting he may attempt to side-track the discussion by becoming involved in an argument, by withdrawing into sullen silence, or by other means of avoidance. It becomes the obligation of all members of the treatment unit to continue to focus on the main issue, the empty feeling. If he cannot learn within the supportive treatment setting to acknowl-edge his personal situation with its associated panic, anxiety, and depression and learn to resolve his difficulties, he will have small chance of altering himself outside of the protected treatment en-vironment. This is true in both the inpatient and the outpatient settings.

Many persons in the counseling role sense the discomfort of the person who is beginning to appraise himself realistically. Staff members become concerned that they are actually hurting the individual and shut off the discussion. In so doing, they con-firm the addict's belief that he is incapable of evaluating himself, bearing discomfort, and changing. In addition, these counselors are treating themselves by avoiding their own discomfort. The *discomfort is mutual, but is a necessary part of the process of change.*

> Rick is a 21-year-old, single college dropout who en-tered the inpatient psychiatric service following a 3-year period of increasingly self-destructive behavior ending in a serious suicide attempt. Although articulate and intelligent, he had been sullen and withdrawn. He either slept or did the bare minimum of activities in the hospital. In a confer-ence with other patients and staff, he stated that his prob-lem was that of being a "con man" who didn't know what was true anymore. His words sounded practiced. They con-tained no feeling. When asked why he wanted the therapist to see him as a con man, he explained that he could change his attitudes to fit the different groups he was with. He knew that he could easily fool people this way and get them to like him.

Rick's aplomb dropped abruptly when he was told that this behavior only indicated that he conned people because he believed that no one would choose to like him or be with him if he were himself. What did he believe was so unlikable about himself? He seemed startled at this direct statement and the question. He was then asked how he had come to believe this. Referring to this first clarification of his behavior, he related how he had tried to comply with changing parental demands. Always attempting to get his parent's affection, he felt that he never quite succeeded. Although real, these incidents had a deceptive quality. He was asked what genuinely hurt him the most. He mentioned that his parents had broken up a homosexual relationship that had developed when he left home for the first time. He angrily criticized his parents for not accepting his open discussion of this relationship. They had always wanted to know what was going on, and he had told them: "Look, they always asked to know what was going on and I tell them. So what do they do? They reject my relationship."

Subsequent comments revealed that Rick never really expected them to accept the relationship. He knew that it would force them to separate from him; this was something he had not been able to do on his own. He wished them to bear the responsibility for his leaving. The therapist pushed further, asking what thoughts were going through his mind. Rick could not say. He was asked to describe his last meeting with his lover. Rick paused, his expression changed, and for the first time he stammered, paused again, blushed, and furiously turned to the doctor saying, "I don't have to tell you." He was then asked what he had been thinking that caused him so much discomfort. He avoided answering, and finally, in a fit of rage, he stated that he had been picturing his lover's body. At this point the therapist's tone shifted, and in a quiet, supportive manner, he asked for the details of the visual memory, the sight, the texture, the smell. With anguish, Rick revealed how he had become furious with his lover and had felt lonely and abandoned. He had wanted to destroy the lover. He was recapturing the sense of emptiness that he had ex-

perienced earlier. The emptiness had covered his own unacceptable hurt and sadistic rage. Both had been avoided in
his previous depression.

Once the pain was out in the open, there was no
longer any need to pressure him. He spoke in a spontaneous, genuine manner about the anguish of losing his lover
and his family, the chronic sense of loneliness that he had
always experienced. His behavior on the unit changed
markedly for the next 3 weeks and he was discharged. He
talked more openly with people and dealt with the issues in
a realistic manner. He approached the interviewing physician and later stated, "You finally got to me. I was so
furious with you I had to do something for myself. I didn't
know that I had so much anger inside me. I had to talk with
you directly. I could no longer avoid the things that hurt
me. You made me look at it, and I couldn't avoid you any
longer. It scared me, but I needed it. I couldn't just lie
back as I have been doing for months. I had to deal with
what was really going on." In the interview, there had been
a steady pressure to face the internal pain and deal with it
openly, instead of avoiding it and reacting impulsively when
avoidance was not possible. At the same time, the presence
and steadiness of the therapist supported the discussion.

This approach worked only because the physician and
other staff members subsequently were not afraid to talk to
Rick about his fear of abandonment and look at it honestly.
Their candor gave him some encouragement that his situation was not hopeless. Outpatient follow-up after 1 year indicates that he is continuing to make substantial gains in
therapy and in his life. Had these issues been skirted because of the patient's initial hostility or a concern about discussing the "nitty-gritty" details of his homosexual experience, he might have continued to believe that his personal
issues were too revolting for others to tolerate and understand.

Action to Avoid Feeling

The addict frequently engages in impulsive actions. Because he cannot bear anxiety, sadness, anger, and humiliation,

he resorts to activities that provide sufficient external stress so as to distract him from his own feelings. As a rule, these actions are poorly planned and usually result in the individual's developing further difficulties within his environment.

Jerry is a 28-year-old factory worker who had been hospitalized for his third overdose suicide attempt. Three times in the 2 years prior to this last admission, he had followed the same pattern, which had led to this hospitalization. On each occasion, he had become involved in gambling with a group of men whom he described as tough and older. His attempts to keep up with them led to increasingly large debts. He began taking household money to cover these expenses. This led to marital disputes in which his wife began ignoring him. In order to punish his wife and get her to respond to him, he openly dated other women. His wife clearly controlled the home, and this was an attempt to build his own sense of self-esteem. Each time this happened, his wife made plans to leave him. At this point, he wrote bad checks and brought money home to pay the debts. When the checks bounced, the merchants or court officers would come to the home seeking to get money for the checks. At this point, he would overdose and be hospitalized.

Each time Jerry was admitted, the hospital staff would try to interrupt the cycle. His parents, however, would pay his debts and talk to his wife about making another attempt to make the marriage work. Each time, she agreed and promised to forget the past behavior if he would only promise not to overdose again. The response of the wife and the parents only supported the recurrence of the ritual. Jerry never had to deal with the real consequences of his behavior. Each action in the self-destructive spiral was the impulsive solution to a previous problem.

The only advantage of such activities is that they distract the person from his own feelings and usually distract those about him so that they don't look at the emotional state that preceded the action. The addict and the observer both agree that these actions are only a temporary solution.

There is a constant necessity to create newer and usually more dangerous diversions.

Other People Are Unreal

Most persons with impulsive personality disorders relate to the individuals around them as if these others are not real people whose needs are as valid as their own. In the patient's view, these others are like cardboard cutouts, placed there to fill out some scene in his life. Other people's wants, needs, wishes, and concerns are unimportant and nonexistent to the person with this disorder. This is evident in the rapid turnover of friends, companions, and spouses.

> As Jack said, "I was really down when she left. I thought I couldn't go on living. The next day, you wouldn't believe it. I met Rachel and, well, that was it. My life was complete again." People are as interchangeable as parts in a machine; each part has a function but one is as good as another.

This "unrealness" is seen even more dramatically in the untroubled commission of violence upon other people.

> Bruce described a random shooting of strangers:
> "I was standing there in the woods shooting at cans when this truck drove by, with a group of men in the back. I thought, wow, I wonder if I can hit one. I just picked up the rifle and *blewee*, that guy jumped. I read in the paper that he had been shot in the shoulder."
> "Well, how did you feel?"
> "Well, you know, that gun really felt great, you know, against my shoulder. It had great balance, it had this special walnut stock—"
> "No, No! What about that man? What about his being shot?"
> "Oh that, nothing special."

Can these printed words convey my incredulity? It is hard to believe people who describe acts of violence toward other human beings without the least concern that the other person also has feelings, hopes, desires. This man was an ordinary person. He was sociable and engaging. He was not crazed. He said he liked people. Yet, he could comfortably shoot another person for no reason and feel no remorse.

Another manifestation of the unreal picturing of other people is seen in preconceived ideas about them and in unrealistic expectations of them. A snap judgment, a first impression is embellished with all of the longings, hopes, and beliefs that these individuals carry within them. They treat their stereotype image as if it represents the whole, real individual: "Women are supposed to care." "Doctors care about people." "Mothers aren't supposed to get tired." When real aspects of the other person's character intrude or an expectation is unmet, the person with the destructive character does not question his original perception. Instead, *he reacts as if the other person purposefully and maliciously deprived him of his rightful expectation. In this context he feels that it is perfectly reasonable to exact whatever revenge he deems necessary.*

No Continuity in Patterns of Events

All events are treated as separate and unrelated. Any similarity between today's crisis, last week's, or last year's is seen as coincidence: "Forget the past; it was yesterday. What does it have to do with today?" When it becomes inescapable that the individual is repeating a pattern of behavior, he usually says, "But that's the way I am, always was, always will be. I can't do anything about it." To accept a continuity in the events of one's life usually leads to the sense of hopelessness. When this occurs, the individual sees it as an externally imposed script: Fate or Society caused it. "What can I do, once a junkie, always a junkie." All of these statements attribute the power and design of personal events to sources outside of the individual.

If one rejects this sense of fatalistic expectation and forces the individual to go over each step in his decisions about particular pieces of behavior, one sees that he has made a series of choices. Evaluating his judgment and the reasons for his choices may lead to the conclusion that he used poor judgment or had other alternatives or resources. People can learn that *they* do make choices (not fate) and that they therefore have the capacity to understand their decisions. Many people have become excited upon seeing this and have actively begun to work out their own repetitious behavior patterns. This sense of excitement usually represents a feeling of relief and freedom from the pervasive sense of doom. If living is indeed a matter of choice, then it is possible for one to learn how to choose differently. If it is a matter of fate, we all are at its mercy.

The stepwise weighing of all the superficially insignificant events involved in a piece of behavior is one method by which the understanding of decisions is gained. In the example of Elton, who had been arrested during a store theft (p. 19), it was this process that allowed us to piece together the events that uncovered his own desire to be relieved of the pressure of taking care of himself. Consequently, he became enthusiastic about learning to make better choices for himself.

Inability to Tolerate Criticism

The person with a character disorder tends to see things in an all-or-none, black-or-white fashion. If he finds one error or deficiency in a person or a program, it is sufficient evidence to discredit it totally. Logically, he is aware that perfection does not exist. However, he needs to find deficiencies in order to support his basic premise—that everyone is the same; there is no hope. He can then validate his position that change is impossible for him. This helps to protect him from self-criticism.

Bill, aged 21, had a history of severe delinquency since age 13. He had been dropped from a drug-treatment program once because of repeated drug use within the institution. Following readmission, he was questioned by his therapy group because he had failed to complete his required work assignment for unit maintenance. He immediately responded in a defensively hostile manner: "I don't care what you guys say. If you don't like it, I'll leave." The therapist intervened and inquired why he would choose to leave the institution and commit himself to a 3-year jail sentence on such minimal provocation. With the same charged emotions, he responded: "They are saying I am nothing—a complete fuck-up—that I don't do anything right."

The specific issue of failure to complete a work assignment was seen as a general and irrevocable character indictment. Bill saw it in this manner because he viewed himself as unalterable. His first statement—"Like it or leave it"— could be translated: "Accept me as I am because I can't change." He could not see a single question or comment about a specific issue as different from a total character assessment, "complete fuck-up."

Such people have little successful accomplishment that would allow them to tolerate criticism. They have nothing to fall back on. It is as if each situation is a new test of their self-esteem. Any criticism has a devastating effect and requires the maximum defensive response. Because the personal image is so fragile, it must be defended at all costs, at all times.

This is an area in which the staff's role model function is important. The capacity of the staff to review their own performance critically and make appropriate changes is a vital factor in this form of treatment. A staff who are defensive and unable to respond to realistic needs for alteration only support the addict's sense of hypocrisy on the part of his alleged helpers. Similarly, a staff who feel overly responsible and guilty about errors set a poor example for the patient.

Inability to Plan

The men frequently talked in terms of long-term objectives: stable homes and families, good jobs. Their conversation had a dreamlike quality, showing no concept of the integral steps necessary to achieve such goals. When they were asked for specific plans, the discussions ended, and the men withdrew from further discussions that challenged the fantasy.

In Lexington, the average maximum duration of any activity not directly organized and maintained by staff members was 2 weeks. Because many of the jobs in the institution were menial and of little personal value, one of the staff proposed that the men refinish furniture as a means of providing useful work and income. The men would have to organize themselves and establish a structure for assigning and carrying out tasks, including purchasing, labor, and sales job assignments.

This idea interested 16 men because they saw it as a way to earn money. Repeatedly, they came to the staff for ideas but did not provide thoughts of their own. In spite of the fact that a room, supplies, and consultation were provided, the number dwindled to 3 men within 2 weeks. Only when a therapist took them into the workshop personally and discussed the plan did they begin work. Many factors contribute to such a situation: resentment, the regressive pull of institutionalization, lack of immediate results. Yet, the men showed a similar lack of capacity for long-range planning while on the streets.

In day-to-day tasks, impulsiveness replaced planning and the weighing of potential outcomes. Underlying this mode of behavior is the individual's sense that for him there is no future. Remembering past experiences of progressively more serious failures, he views himself as powerless and directed by forces that he cannot influence.

Inability to Delay Gratification

This is a corollary of the inability to plan. Demands must be met immediately because there is no belief that the future will provide better results. The concept of coming months and years is vague, and the focus is only on the present. The past often is too painful to review. As a result of these factors, failure to meet a demand immediately often results in massive emotional responses.

Trent had been in Lexington for 1 day when he demanded to see the therapist in order to be discharged.

Once seen, he did not want to discuss the reasons for his sudden decision. It was pointed out that his addiction was of long duration and that his 1 day in the center had neither given him time either to be physiologically withdrawn nor to evaluate the program in terms of his own needs. He continued to demand that he be discharged immediately. The fact that he had agreed with the judge to a period of 14 days made no difference.

The unit policy of asking all men to wait 14 days before leaving in order to make a more realistic appraisal of the center was also explained. Trent had been aware of these conditions prior to admission, but this in no way influenced his thinking. It was pointed out that he was free to walk out the door at any time; however, the institution would not certify that he had received an adequate evaluation. If he left prior to the 14 days without such sanction, he would have violated the agreement with the court and would possibly be subject to legal action. If he could wait out the minimum time, he could certainly exercise his right to leave. Again and again, he demanded that he be given the appropriate discharge papers certifying a complete evaluation. He gave no explanation and continued to state, "I just want to go." He became more enraged and refused to deal with any of the issues, either personal or legal. After 3 days he left explaining that he had not known what he was getting into, that he would rather take his chances with the court than wait out the 9 remaining days.

Entitlement

This attitude pervades many of the addict's interactions with institutions, professional persons, and family members. He speaks and acts as if it is reasonable to expect that he receive some material good or benefit that was never promised.

Randy, aged 26, had a hand and wrist deformity that slightly limited his function. It had resulted from a self-inflicted injury many years before. During his physical examination on admission, he began questioning the physician as to when the corrective surgery would be done and what were the qualifications of the surgeon. He was told that a physician from a nearby university medical center could be consulted and possibly corrective surgery could be done. It was explained that the treatment center's facilities served emergencies only.

Furious, Randy insisted that this was a government-supported hospital, and wasn't the government supposed to provide *whatever* he needed? When asked what had led him to expect this, he would only say, "That's the way it is supposed to be."

In his personal dealings, the addict demonstrates the same attitudes. Minimal provocation entitles him to a maximum response. It is someone else's responsibility to provide for his needs. His only role is that of the wrongly deprived individual who has earned the right to some form of restitution.

Frequently, a more subtle version of this attitude emerges, and the staff members find themselves beginning to feel uncomfortable in saying "no" to what is basically an unreasonable request.

The individual may set up the situation by calling himself inept: "You know, I am just a junkie." He then portrays the staff person as an abundant source of necessary goods and concern. By establishing these roles, he plays upon the staff member's guilt and discomfort at refusing to grant the request and further implies that the staff member is not fulfilling his or her role as a helper.

Some of the men were standing near the soda machine at Lexington, when a staff member put in some coins to get a drink. Josh began telling her that he had not heard from home in a long time and therefore could not buy cigarettes or soda. She glanced about uncomfortably as he spoke. He then asked her to buy him a drink: "It is a small thing. You're working and can easily afford it. What can I do? I don't have any money." She stammered and blushed as she tried to say no gracefully. He responded, "That's great, here I ask a little thing from someone who is supposed to care and she says no." He continued his harangue

until she left in a huff saying, "All you fellows are alike."
Josh picked up his newly acquired tape recorder and shirts
and walked off, cursing her with a smile on his face.

No Experience Bearing Anxiety or Discomfort

The men and women at the center demonstrated little ability to put up with physical pain, emotional frustration, depression, or anxiety. They demanded immediate relief, which had to come from someone else. At Lexington, men frequently forgot dental appointments that had been scheduled because of serious dental problems. It was quite common that shortly after the forgotten appointment, the individual demanded that he be seen immediately because the pain had intensified. Following an extraction, men refused aspirin or Darvon because codeine was the only medicine that would *completely* relieve the pain. There was no idea of bearing some discomfort.

Clearly, a number of the traits previously discussed are included here: inability to delay gratification, poor planning, impulsiveness. Because the sufferer believes that the future provides no hope of relief, he must focus on the present. These individuals need to be educated *in a noncritical way* to expect discomfort and learn to bear it. Their self-esteem is increased when they can see a reason for tolerating discomfort and when they find they are able to do so. This is not an invitation for sadistic or masochistic interactions. The capacity to bear some discomfort with a clear goal in mind is part of the process of maturation.

When an individual reports that he has successfully managed a stressful situation without resorting to his usual self-destructive means, the question should be: What internal resources did he use to cope with the situation? This allows him to begin to see that he has previously ignored strength and abilities that he may be able to call upon in the future. *It is of paramount importance that the individual define his internal strengths or he is liable to see a particular success as a result of institutionalization or association with the people around him.* He must learn to view his success as a consequence of personal resources, not random chance. Failure to see this will further his belief that today's success was only a temporary respite in his chronic downhill course.

If he defines his inner assets, they will become available in the future. It is in this kind of situation that he can begin to view himself as having a positive role in the direction of his life. In this way, he can begin to learn that discomfort is bearable and a prerequisite for growth.

Gabriella, a married mother of three with a history of repeated overdoses and self-inflicted lacerations, was seen in a psychiatric clinic for recurrent depressions. Each week, she came to the office with a bona fide crisis. Each time, the therapist quelled his own impulse to reassure her and obtain relief for her by calling social agencies that could deal with the current crisis. Instead, he responded in a quiet but firm voice, "Well, what are *you* going to do about it?" Initially, she responded furiously, "What am *I* going to do? You are the doctor, you are supposed to tell me."

In one instance, she was facing eviction from her apartment that afternoon. After failing to get the therapist to intervene, she said, "Well, I could burn all the furniture." The therapist responded by nodding and apparently writing her suggestion down. Infuriated, she screamed, "I could push it all out the window or get drunk." He nodded and wrote it down. Finally, she said, "I could call some friends and borrow some money and probably pay the rent." He wrote that down too. After noting each suggestion, he questioned the patient as to its merit. Burning, drinking, or destroying the furniture the patient readily discarded. She ridiculed the therapist's serious treatment of these suggestions (although they were in fact consistent with some of her earlier behavior).

By evaluating each suggestion, even though it was given sarcastically, the patient was forced to evaluate her plans and pick the one that had potentially the greatest chance for success. By repeating this process in each crisis, the patient gradually learned that she could devise her own solutions to a problem by evaluating the options and the consequences. She even learned to anticipate the problems and apply her experience when dealing with other issues. When therapy was terminated a year later, she reviewed it and said, "I guess the best thing I learned from you was, 'So, what are you going to do about it?' You really meant I could do something, that I didn't need to get an answer from you." She ended by noting, "This reality you've taught me about, it's a pain in the ass. At least I can do something about it!"

Self-Destruction

The person with a destructive character disorder is always self-destructive. Whatever the means—drugs, alcohol, repeated suicide gestures, prostitution, habitual criminal activity—the result is that he or she must constantly pay a price for transient relief of internal pressure. Underlying this pattern, there always seems to be a sense of guilt and worthlessness.

Close to three-quarters of the men who completed the program at Lexington gave a history of early parental injunctions with alternatives clearly defined: "If you don't listen to me and do what I say, you'll wind up a no account thief like your father." "The worst thing that could happen would be for you to wind up a thief and a junkie."

With amazing regularity, the men chose these alternatives. A typical history would involve a family from which the father had been absent since the patient was 5 years old. The son would develop close ties with the mother. He would go to school, attend church, and avoid the delinquent group of children prohibited by his mother. His reward would be praise coupled with an admonition: "Watch out or you will be like your father."

Around 13, the boy's behavior would begin to change and the mother's admonitions would increase. He would speak of being independent, being a man, and not needing his mother. His independent behavior would invariably follow the pattern of his mother's admonition:

1. Hal said, "It was amazing. Mother would say you don't know what you're doing. If you go out tonight, you will be arrested. I would say, 'I know what I am doing. I can take care of myself, Ma.' You know, that is just what happened. I would always get arrested. I don't know how she knew." When asked, "Who would bail you out?" he said, "She did, of course!"

2. Rudy had been an A student in high school. During the adolescent years, his severely abusive father paid little attention to his athletic or academic success but frequently told the boy, "The lowest things are dope fiends and thieves. Don't you ever go in for that stuff." Rudy reflected later, "I can't understand it. I became both."

3. Obie remembered thinking about his mother's injunction against thieves while committing a burglary. "I paused and thought about what she had said and I said to myself, 'Ah, fuck it, the hell with her, the hell with me. I'll show her.'" He then proceeded to finish the burglary and get arrested. He showed her! Interestingly, had he not paused, he would probably not have been arrested.

Such persons act as if there are only two choices in life. Both have been defined by some family member. The first choice is compliance with what is defined by the family as the positive role. Fitting into this role continues to provide the individual with a parent–child relationship. The second role, or the deviant position, provides a posture that is called independence by the patient. During adolescence, he opts for the second role since being a child is no longer acceptable.

The first position allows the individual to receive some affection and care but necessitates giving up growth, independence, and separation from his family. For males with only a mother in the home, it is tantamount to voluntary emasculation. The second position allows the person to express his aggression toward the family member indirectly without danger of rupturing their tie. His deviant behavior confirms the parent's earlier statement that if he fails to follow a particular course, he will turn out badly. In effect, he says, "Yes, Mother and Father, you were right." He verbally says, "I am independent; I don't need your help," but behaviorally he tells them, "You must care for me." By this, he means buy him drugs, bail him out, care for him when he is sick. When confronted with such an analysis, the men usually responded, "I didn't ask her to bail me out." Yet, they did not fail to notify the family of their need for help. Thus, these individuals could be verbally independent while behaving quite dependently.

Because an individual has not overtly requested a particular form of help, he acts as if he bears no responsibility for another person's response to his presentation of himself as helpless and needy. This seems to be part of a functional system in which family and patient fail to separate adequately. He and his family (or the family substitute) go on in this seemingly endless duet. The addict denies responsibility for the family's anguish because he did not plan to cause any discomfort. The family continues to rescue him and promotes the idea that, in fact, he is a little child who must be cared for. Neither has to deal with the painful issues of mature separation and personal responsibility.

This system satisfies each party: the addict can be rebellious and show his anger without threatening the dependent relationship; the family continues to feel they must take care of the little child who has never grown up and still needs them.

The addict frequently acts as though he belongs to a particular member of the family. He does not focus on the injury to himself but only on its effect upon the person with whom he feels connected. Toward this person, he feels an anger related to his sense that he needs the other person to survive. This is a feeling that he resents and tries to deny through his verbal statements and behavior. Like the proverbial poor relative, he silently curses the better-endowed benefactor.

Many of the men are intelligent, skilled, and articulate, yet they never develop a viable alternative to the two positions outlined by the family. To do so would, in effect, be saying, "*You* were wrong. I am able to take care of myself without you." Then the addict would risk the loss of the relationship, which he perceives as being conditional. He hears the message, "I will love you and care for you only if you choose one of the two alternatives I have outlined." The loss of this affection and protection would leave the individual potentially alone to fend for himself. Having received an inadequate experience in terms of love, affection, and growth assistance in the family previously, the individual in this bind is hesitant to part with the little he does receive in order to face what he believes will be a lonely, more painful existence. As one man put it, "Better to be the black sheep, than no sheep." Since he does not feel adequate on his own, he will not hazard such a move toward real independence. Separation from the real or the fantasized family relationships is frequently equated with death. Feeling himself connected to and dependent upon others, the addict may injure himself as a means of inflicting pain upon those other people. At times, the self-destructiveness has a quality of penance and guilt reduction. The self-destructiveness always seems to be related to significant people in the patient's life. It does not matter whether they are present or absent. The patient carries them about internally all of the time.

When the primary family is gone, wives and institutions are selected as surrogates. The individual carries an internal image of the missing person. He continues the relationship with the missing person in behavior by repeating the same patterns of activity. To change would mean breaking a tie with the lost person. Obie dealt with the internal image of his absent mother when he paused while committing the robbery and relived his dialogue with her (p. 64). By committing the crime he once again demonstrated his independence.

> Doris was a compliant and shy young woman who never rebelled in any way against the pattern of dependent behavior she had evolved with her mother. She stayed home and spent time with her mother and assisted her in household chores. Her reward was a constant shower of praise that was contingent upon her complying with her mother's wishes.
>
> When Doris was 12, her mother became promiscuous with older men and started going to nightclubs with them. She began drinking excessively, made several suicide at-

tempts, and saw a psychiatrist. During this time, Doris
tried to fill her mother's role in the home and care for the
younger children. She could not acknowledge her disappointment and anger toward her mother. As her mother became progressively more erratic, Doris began to pray that
"God would take her." Several weeks later, her mother
died from an overdose of barbiturates and alcohol.

Following her mother's death, Doris became promis-
cuous, preferring older men and frequenting the same
nightclubs as her mother. She began using alcohol and barbiturates, made several suicide attempts, and sought help
from the same psychiatrist her mother had seen. She began
wearing her mother's clothes.

In therapy, the evidence of the rage toward her
mother began mounting and she became overtly psychotic
for a short time. She spoke to her mother's picture in her
wallet as if she were her constant companion. Without her,
she felt she could not survive. Her reenactment of her
mother's tragic course was based upon a longing to return
to her and guilt over the thought that her wish had killed
her. She gradually began to explore the love and affection
she had for her mother, as well as the anger and hurt. Her
mother had encouraged Doris to stay home and be like her
or face an emotional abandonment similar to her mother's
treatment of her father. She had complied with her threat
because it meant never being apart. Then, her mother
reneged upon their agreement, by dying.

Doris's story highlights in an extreme fashion the
dangers underlying the excessive and intense parent–child
relationship seen in many addicted individuals. Separation
from a parent with whom one has not been able to resolve
basic issues of love, aggression, and growth can seem impossible. The separation becomes intimately linked with destruction—one's own destruction and/or the destruction of
one's parent.

Examples of Depression

The preceding discussion of character traits implies that a
pervasive and overwhelming depression underlies the destructive personality disorder. Wherever we have succeeded in get-

ting an addict to relinquish his blaming-the-world stance (projective defense) and actions of avoidance and distraction, a devastating depression has emerged. For example, one patient said, "My God, if I were to listen to you and think of all the stuff I have done, I couldn't like myself. I would have to kill myself. It makes me feel I'm nothing."

During one 10-month period in Lexington, 35% of the men sought out staff members because of depression following a comprehensive evaluation conference on their lives and behavior. These conferences included detailed investigation of the person's growth, development, and family relationships. Following this the unit staff reviewed the man's behavior within the institution. All of this was conducted with the patient present. There then ensued a 1½-hour psychiatric interview. A definite attempt was made to see patterns of behavior, to interpret defenses, and to confront the person with his role in the development of his current status. The tone was nonpunitive and an attitude developed that encouraged the man to look at his behavior as having meaning.

When men sought help after such conferences, they complained of depression specifically relating to the points of view presented to them. During these subsequent sessions, they were particularly troubled by the repetition in their destructive patterns. Previously, they had seen their acts as single incidents not connected to each other in a meaningful way. This view had protected them from a depression caused by seeing the ongoing consistency of their destructive behavior.

Spontaneous descriptions of themselves as isolated and depressed during the evaluation for admission were given by 28% of the men. They thought this accounted for their initial and continued use of drugs. The depression was not a time-limited feeling. The men spoke of their lives as always having been hopeless. Frequently, there was a turning point when their lives went from bad to worse. This was usually associated with the loss of a fantasy of restitution. For example, an addict may have thought, "When I am bigger, I will put the family together again; mother will return; someday father will stop drinking and care for me." When such a fantasy is lost, the individual experiences a depression characterized by: (1) a sense of personal worthlessness and emptiness, and a belief that improvement is impossible; (2) a fear that close relationships are destructive; and (3) indecisiveness and lack of motivation toward any goal. There seems to be no use to anything. They seem to be stuck in time, unable to move forward with their own lives. They live in a state of existential paralysis.

Even after detoxification, these patients were listless. Aside from an appearance of anger, their tone of voice and their facial expressions hardly changed. They showed no sexual interest except in terms of using women to prove their manliness to other men. Their humor was based upon sadistic humiliation of others. Surprisingly enough, they maintained a vague delusion that "In spite of my past history, something will happen and things will turn out all right."

> Zeb, 32, is a divorced high school dropout who had entered the Lexington center for his third time. Having stated early in this stay that he felt his situation was hopeless and that he believed he would return to drugs, he later said, "I know it looks that way [hopeless]; I know it sounds that way [hopeless]. My words say it, and I say it, but that isn't the case. I know somehow it will be different." The delusion involved a desperate and unrealistic belief that in spite of the reality of the situation, everything would be "okay."

Hope is a necessary human attribute. It is most useful when tied to realistic possibilities. In neurotic depressions, the patients reproach themselves. For the criminal or addict in this situation, the admission of one error is equivalent to a total and irrevocable judgment of himself. For this reason, he uses all of the defenses at his disposal to avoid acknowledging any error or any involvement in making a mistake: "It was all someone else's fault. I had nothing to do with it." Thus, expressions of self-reproach were absent. Yet, the punishing self-reproach was evident in self-destructiveness and side comments: "I know I ain't worth nothing."

Direct references to suicidal thoughts or plans, present in neurotic depressions, are denied by these impulsive people but again are repeatedly evidenced in self-destructive behavior. *Thus, the depression experienced by the person with a self-destructive personality is characterized by the acting out of feelings of depression without his conscious acknowledgment.* The task of treatment is to help the individual become aware of his depression so that he will no longer need to seek a solution through destructive behavior. Because the individual is not aware of the feelings of depression, the most accurate appraisal of his emotional state comes from observation of his behavior, not his words. It is obvious that people who feel good about themselves do not destroy themselves!

CHAPTER 4

Developmental Defect

This chapter deals with two crucial issues. One is my formulation of the origin of the problem of impulsive behavior. The second point is an outgrowth of the first and represents a means of viewing impulsive behavior that does not get mired in the specifics of one particular diagnostic entity versus another. Many important concepts from ego and developmental psychology are left out, blurred, or lumped together for the purpose of simplification and clarity. Sophisticated readers may appropriately object to this. I would ask their forbearance as the book is written to convey views and concepts to less experienced people from a variety of backgrounds.

The formulation that is most helpful to me in understanding the origin of impulsive behavior came about through repeated interviews, conferences, and therapy experiences with approximately 500 patients at all of the institutions previously mentioned, as well as in my private practice.

A review of the history with these patients revealed similar experiences. Many times the pattern of events did not emerge until months after treatment began, when particular events and feelings were remembered.

From birth until some time between ages 3–7 years, the typical patient lived in a relatively comfortable personal state.

Even if the home and family suffered from problems of sickness, alcoholism, emotional absence, etc., there was a relative stability in the chaos or deprivation. One person, usually the mother, but possibly an aunt or grandparent, became the person upon whom the developing individual focused all of his hopes for gratification and satisfaction. Between ages 3 and 7, this person suddenly changed or was lost to the patient. This abrupt loss of the potential for satisfaction and nurturance became the focal point of development. The loss may have occurred through death, illness, divorce, alcoholism, or a severe emotional withdrawal by the physically present individual. The pain and rage of this loss created a sense of panic and hopelessness within the developing individual. Frequently, the nurturant person had become so crucial because he or she seemed to represent the only potential for relief from the other painful realities and developmental conflicts. This loss and the subsequent panic led to a developmental defect in the individual's capacity to handle emotions that trigger off a renewed sense of the original panic. When they experience this panic, they react impulsively.

In order to develop this concept more clearly, it may be helpful to review briefly some aspects of child development.

Normal Development

Ordinarily, children develop in an environment that tends to nurture them and caters to their needs from birth until approximately age 1–2. When children start walking, certain behavioral limits are imposed. Similarly, early attempts at self-feeding and food preferences may provoke the imposition of behavioral limits. Usually around age 2, several significant changes occur. The development of speech shifts the emphasis from behaviorally imposed limits to a combination of verbal and behavioral expectations and limits. The demand for bowel and bladder control involves language, impulse control, and expectations. The struggle over expectations, independence, dependence, and limits extends to the areas of independent feeding, dressing, sharing, etc.

Parents use a number of methods to help the child develop in these areas. Frequently, the struggle causes the parent to become angry, and he or she transiently withdraws approval and affection. Such withdrawal may result in a reactive anger on the part of the child, which is then followed by a panic-motivated attempt to regain the withheld affection. These brief periods of emotional separation followed by a reunion with the nurturing parent are frequently coupled with an attempt to please the parent by fulfilling the expectations.

In addition to emotional separation, the child learns to tolerate physical separations from the parents. Visiting playmates and preschool nursery experiences are followed by the entrance into grammar school. By this time, the child has developed sufficient autonomy and impulse control to be able to function independently of parental input for short periods. For this sequence to develop, the child has repeatedly had the reassurance that brief separations from the parent are always followed by a reunion. The parent does not disappear forever!

Concomitant with the preschool and early grammar-school period, the child goes through a time when he or she seeks to win the exclusive attention of the parent of the opposite sex. This three-way struggle among the child and the two parents (Oedipal phase) usually resolves as the child finds that it is impossible to displace one parent's affection from the other. This necessary injury to the child's self-esteem is diminished by valuing and identifying assets in the former rival. In order to win someone like the desired parent in the future, the child tries to become like the parent of the same sex.

This process is usually diminished by age 7–9. Energy from these earlier conflicts is diverted to learning skills and talents until the adolescent period. In these early years, the emphasis shifts from behavior and the modulation of the expression of strong emotions to understanding and dealing with verbally expressed feelings. By age 9, the child has developed semi-independent mechanisms for coping with strong emotions. The parental role shifts to meeting more complex and subtle changes in personal development. Some parents put it succinctly when they say, "Now I can talk to him, I don't have to sit on him all the time." For a few years, the child accepts the parents' expectations and view of the world. There is still a need for parental reinforcement and support but less need for direct intervention. This period of relative calm during development ends during preadolescence and adolescence.

During the adolescent period, the developing adult contends with changes in body physiology and proportion, as well as a reexamination of previously accepted beliefs. Part of the earlier acceptance of parental attitudes is related to the state of dependence upon available adults for basic life needs. Another factor in this early acceptance is the ability of the important adults to enforce their will physically upon the child. During adolescence, the relative importance of both of these factors diminishes.

When the adolescent phase of development proceeds in an adequate manner, the maturing person struggles with himself and his parents as he tests and reevaluates previously unquestioned premises. Some of these previously accepted beliefs are found to be empty and hypocritical. Much of the anger and frustration of adolescence represents the loss of the protective fantasies of childhood and the gradual anguished acceptance of the uncertainty and imperfection of the real or adult world. Once again, there is a preoccupation with strong emotions, impulse-control expectations, conscience, and separation from family.

This process is aided by the adolescent's realization that he can have an effect upon the course of his own life. Neither is he completely powerless, nor is he or his parents all powerful. Another factor in this process is the ongoing availability of parents or their substitutes who will maintain a relationship, even when they are needed in a new and different manner. Thus, the young adult who no longer needs his parents in the same way is reassured by finding that the separation is not total. A comfortable, more equal relationship begins developing in the early and mid 20s.

What happens when these briefly outlined developmental steps are interrupted before reaching their natural conclusion?

Loss

The impulse-ridden individuals described in this book have not had the parental or family availability and interest outlined above. Data from a number of clinical experiences indicated the occurrence of developmental problems during the early years of growth in the patients under treatment.

1. There was the need in treatment to establish behavioral limits and expectations out of proportion for adults of their age. The therapist had to be prepared to demonstrate the capacity to exercise controls in a physical manner more appropriate for children between ages 2 and 7. These individuals had not reached a point in their development where verbal interaction had become the ally of their own internalized controls. This fact correlated well with the period in normal development when children are verbal but need the external reinforcement of adults to maintain their own development capacity to control the expression of feelings and impulses.

2. The review of the 400 men at Lexington and the 65 male and female so-called borderline patients on the psychiatric inpatient service showed a consistent, significant alteration in the family status between ages 3 and 7 years. Death, illness, alcoholism, divorce, or a marked alteration in the emotional availability of one or both parents due to emotional illness occurred in almost all cases during the period from age 3–7 in the child's life. In those instances in which the instability and emotional unavailability within the family was resolved, it was not until the patient's mid teens. The patient effectively suffered a crucial and frequently permanent loss of emotional input from the parents after a period of relative stability.

3. Following the emotional loss of one parent, the child frequently turned to the remaining parent, who was usually impaired by his own sense of loss. Many times the female children

were sought out by their fathers and developed incestuous relationships. Male children continued angry and provoking behavior through grammar school or experienced an uncontrolled re-emergence of it during early adolescence. Of the 45 borderline patients from the inpatient psychiatric service, 16 (15 women, 1 man) had experienced incestuous relations with a parent. Many of these patients reported genital manipulation and contact with the parents beginning at age 5–6. In their adult sexual experience, these individuals preferred oral sexual experiences to genital contact. They described these as filling a sense of personal emptiness. *However, the sexual experiences were far less important to these people than the aspects of sexual behavior that involved cuddling, caressing, being held, and not being left alone at night.* Such nocturnal fears and needs for closeness and comfort are characteristic of these early years. *Thus, these people traded intimacy for the needed comfort and protection from fearful anxiety.*

4. Intensive psychotherapy with individuals who have experienced incest as children consistently shows that where incest has occurred, the individuals involved show little capacity to believe that there are realistic limits to any situation. Their experience has proved that there are no limits. There had been no boundary to this stringent cultural taboo. How could they then believe that there really are other limits? If parents don't control impulses, does anyone? They all showed a belief in the magical and omnipotent qualities of their own thoughts and fantasies. This related directly to the incest. They remembered wishes and fantasies for intense and intimate experiences with their parents that had been later realized. They had come to believe that their wishes for an intimate relationship had been powerful enough to cause the parent to act. This reinforced the normal childhood beliefs in the power of magic, thoughts, and wishes. Such beliefs in magic and wish fulfillment are also consistent with the age 3–7. The wish fulfillment, not only frightened these people but caused them to feel guilty and responsible for the actions of their parents.

The high incidence of incest is mentioned only to indicate

the amount of desperation these individuals experience because of the parental loss and the lengths to which they will go in order to hold onto the remaining but impaired parent. Many others, in their desperation, became compliant until the problems of separation and loss were rekindled during adolescence. This involvement with the remaining parent, whether through compliance or through an active struggle, serves as an attempt to regain the nurturing lost parent. The young woman who has sexual experiences with her father as a means of being held close and avoiding loneliness seeks the same thing as the delinquent who is caught and forces his parents to bail him out, get him a lawyer, and escort him to court. They both engage the parent or parent substitute in an intimate relationship.

The nature of the loss may vary. The mother or the mothering adult may become physically ill, die, become depressed and withdrawn, or develop alcoholism or drug abuse. Some mothers become angry, sullen, withdrawn, and depressed when they are abandoned by their husbands. Other mothers can meet the early, more easily managed nurturing demands of the infant. They are overwhelmed by the more complex needs of the verbal and resistant child.

Compounding the loss is the denial of it. A father's abandonment and the mother's subsequent depression frequently go unexplained. The child is thought to be too young to understand, or the parent is attempting to deny his or her distress by overtly ignoring the loss. For these reasons, the child is given no explanation of the remaining parent's emotional alteration. Without clarification, the child is bewildered. He feels a distress that is poorly defined. He notes a difference in one or both parents but is unable to get them to explain it.

Repeatedly, the same events were noted. Relatively stable supports were available until sometime between ages 3 and 7. During that critical period when independence, separation, impulse control, self-esteem, and conscience were developing, a significant change occurred in the potentially nurturing parent (mainly the mother). The developmental process was interrupted as the child experienced a confusing sense of abandonment. Subsequently, he experienced inconsistent expectations and limits, parental unavailability, and negative role models (alcoholic, angry, abusive, or indifferent parents). These contrasted with the expectations of and relationship to the previously available person. In many instances, the idealized and lost person only represented the hope for an alternative to the other emotionally deficient adults. By focusing on the potentially gratifying person, the child had ignored the other deprivations.

The anguished and confused child attempted to build a new equilibrium with the available but frequently impaired parent. At the same time, the child experienced an inordinate sense of guilt and responsibility for the altered family situation. Attempts to please and regain the parental affection alternated with outbursts of anger. The demands of adolescence caused a reemergence of the pain of this initial loss. The original sense of guilt and responsibility were coupled with a sense of worthlessness. This sense of worthlessness was a consequence of the initial loss: *"If I were a good and worthwhile child, you would not have abandoned me."* Thus the pain of adolescence was compounded by the early loss and guilt. Each new experience presented the individual with a renewed sense of the original loss. A cycle developed in which situations easily triggered the initial panic over loss, the sense of worthlessness, and the impulse-ridden outrage.

Reactions to the Loss

The core of depression referred to earlier reflects the inner turmoil (unresolved conflict) about the early loss and its causes. There are clear elements of guilt, feelings of responsibility for parental loss and of worthlessness, fears of internal impulses, and panic. The recurrent behavioral cycle represents an attempt to rework the original situation by creating analogous ones. As children play out painful experiences in their games, over and over, so do their older counterparts. It is an attempt to relieve the guilt and resolve the original doubts about one's basic value and the nature of one's drives. A number of men report their prison experiences as emotionally relieving. They are (1) contained (impulses allegedly controlled); (2) punished (guilt is relieved); (3) defined as bad (good–bad uncertainty temporarily resolved); (4) nurtured (food, shelter, clothing provided) without having to ask (asking requires acknowledging a need and dependency as well as hazarding a refusal); and (5) noticed and acknowledged (one's presence, comings, and goings are carefully monitored). The prison experience clearly contains many other, more visible and brutally uncomfortable aspects, yet these basic psychological needs are also met.

One might ask why the child sees himself as responsible for parental loss, absence, or indiscretion. Because young children are so totally dependent upon their parents for survival, they find it too disruptive to believe that their parents might be seriously deficient or wrong. In order to minimize their own anxiety, children maintain the fantasy that their parents know and understand everything. To protect and maintain this myth of parental infallibility, the young child resorts to mental gymnastics. Although a child may verbally reject a parental view as unfair or wrong, at the same time he begins an inward search to find where the parent is right.

If a child fails to receive adequate love and affection, which include reasonable expectations and limits, he painfully assumes that there is something wrong or bad within himself. If he experiences emotions or needs that his parents fail to acknowledge or fulfill, he assumes that he contains unacceptable (bad) feelings and needs. He comes to believe that his parents, in their wisdom, see something about him that he cannot see. As a consequence, they rightly withhold their love and affection and withdraw from him. Such a conclusion on the part of the child is frequently followed by overt acts of deviant behavior. These acts (1) attract the parents' attention (restore the lost person); (2) require punishment for being bad (thereby relieve guilt); (3) express some of the rage and hurt; and finally, (4) confirm the alleged wisdom of the parent who supposedly perceives the inherently bad traits.

Terry reflected some of these thoughts in the following ruminative sequence. "Man, I was free as a bird. My parents never cared if I went to school or not" (*loud, bravado*). (*Pause.*) "I don't know whether they cared about anything I did" (*spoken softly in a distracted manner*). (*Pause.*) "What was wrong with me that they didn't care? Parents are supposed to care!" (*spoken angrily*). "I guess I just wasn't worth it" (*spoken with resignation*). "Shit! There's nothing wrong with me" (*the self-doubt acknowledged and denied*). The subsequent emergence of his depression focused on these very issues.

The lack of necessary structure, attention, and positive responses from the parents on a consistent basis during childhood result in the individual's making certain assumptions about himself: (1) "There is something *irrevocably* wrong about me." (2) "I am different and separate from others." (3) "I am therefore unlovable." (4) "My parents were right in not caring for me."

All of these conclusions are a means of avoiding a basic, more painful reality. Briefly stated it is this. Through no fault of the child's the parent did not have the capacity to provide for the particular need of the child. The capacity to meet the need was absent in the parent, not purposely withheld! *It was not there!* The repetition of the childhood response to loss through self-destructive behavior frequently represents the inability to give up the wish for gratification from the original source or its substitutes.

George's mother had abandoned him at age 6 when his father died. He was raised by his grandparents. He sought psychotherapy during his early 20s when repeated episodes of depression, drug abuse, and fighting led to pressure from his grandparents and the law to seek help. During 4 years of twice-weekly psychotherapy, he repeatedly uncovered memories of these early experiences. Each time a memory was recovered, there were several weeks of anger and destructive behavior. Some 2½ years after therapy had begun, there were several weeks of anger focusing upon his mother's abandoning him to his grandparents. She had been hospitalized with a depression following her husband's death and never recovered her former state. Finally, the therapist said, "You know it wasn't your fault that your mother didn't show more attention to your needs. She just didn't have it to give. It just wasn't there." George yelled that he couldn't stand hearing that. It was too painful. "She had to have it! Mothers are supposed to!" There was, however, no self-destructive behavior after this session. For the next 6 weeks, George noted a sense of relief and anguished sadness related to the issue of parental inadequacy. Much of the rest of his therapy experience focused on the sadness he felt about the inability of his parents to meet his legitimate needs.

The depression, as defined above, is a constant experience of the addict. The sense of being worthless and different from all other people is like a raw nerve that is easily touched. It is a trigger. It is this sensitivity that accounts for the self-destructive panic. When his worthlessness is touched, the individual reacts without thought of the consequences. The panic demands an immediate response, immediate relief. *This panic state and the inability to cope with it represent the central defect in the individual's emotional makeup.* The experience of this panic state overrides all self-observation, plans, hopes, guilt, or resolve.

This panic state is a reexperiencing of the initial sense of loss and personal worthlessness that first occurred in childhood. The totality of this experience leads the individual to respond in a seemingly exaggerated way. Thus, relatively minor events may bring about furious responses.

Rick described such an outburst. He was at a party sitting with a friend when a nearby drunk began to say over and over, "Jerk! Jerk!" Rick told him to stop, but the man continued and now directed his drunken murmur at Rick. Suddenly Rick erupted. He smashed a bottle and jammed it in the man's face. Rick said he would have killed him if his friend had not pulled him off. At first, he stated that he knew he had a bad temper but didn't know why he had attacked the stranger. He could not blame it on alcohol because he had not yet been served. He even noted that the man was just a harmless, annoying drunk like many others he had seen. As the discussion continued, Rick remembered that the words and taunting quality were the same as those used by his mother. As he said this, he became choked with rage about "that bitch." Allegedly, economic privation had led the family to break up when he was four. When the family was reconstituted years later, he was not included for several years. All of the other children had returned home. Whether the facts were accurate or not, Rick always responded to the words *jerk* or *stupid* by becoming enraged. Even the inference of such comments caused him to react. They reflected his doubts about himself. During the conference, he said, "Until now, I never realized how that is always there in my mind. I never stop thinking about it—how she left me and taunted me. I always hear that sing-song: 'jerk, jerk. You're nothing but a jerk!' "

If one accepts the concept that chronically impulsive behavior has its root in a developmental defect in the capacity to handle certain emotional states, then one can begin to conceptualize impulsive character disorders according to the way the individual pathologically manages these emotions.

Using a drawing system that is developed further later in the book (Chapter 7), one can visualize several forms of impulsive character disorders.

Figure 1 is comprised of a number of elements:

Part 1. This rectangle represents the impulsive individual. Part 1A represents the way in which the individual believes that he appears to those about him. It also includes aspects of himself that others might see and that the individual does not.

In Part 1B, the broken vertical lines represent the individual's defenses (psychological protective maneuvers) against his own awareness of negative beliefs and doubts about himself. The lines are broken as a way of representing the inconsistency and inadequacy of these defenses.

Part 1C represents the individual's private view of himself, which contains the individual's doubts and beliefs about himself.

The Impulsive Individual

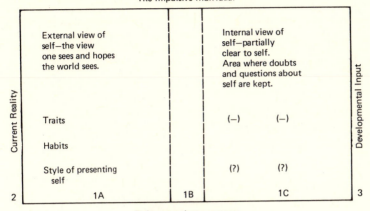

Figure 1

Part 1C does *not* correspond to the concept of the unconscious (the area of one's psychological makeup that contains issues, feelings, and memories that are out of one's awareness). Issues and emotions in area 1C are constantly close to the individual's awareness. They are preconscious or moderately suppressed (intentionally put aside as when the individual says, "I don't let myself think about that.").

Part 2. This is the area of current experience or reality.

Part 3. This is the area of developmental input, where growth issues and experiences contribute to the premises, doubts, and negative beliefs that the individual contains within himself (Part 1C).

Figure 2 begins on the right and progresses to the left. Starting with (1) parental inconsistency and abandonment (real and emotional), the individual comes to assume that he is (2) wrong and bad, thus (3) causing and justifying the initial parental abandonment (reverse arrow). The belief that one is bad leads to a sense of (4) not deserving (guilt and conscience formation).

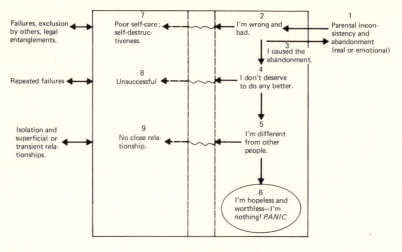

Figure 2

This, in turn, leads to a sense of (5) being irrevocably different and therefore set apart from others. This issue is frequently worked and reworked in the rhetorical argument that impulsive people conduct among themselves as they try to prove that no one is really any different from themselves. This sense of apartness, however, leads to the conclusion of (6) total and abysmal hopelessness and worthlessness—a sense of being nothing. When the individual reaches this conclusion, he is overwhelmed by the anxiety and panic previously mentioned.

The beliefs about being bad, not deserving, and different can be seen as partially expressed (broken arrow) through apparent character traits and recurrent life experiences (7,8,9). When a real-life event triggers off the sequence of "I'm bad" → "I'm undeserving" → "I'm different" → "I'm nothing," one can then observe the emergence of the panic. I have observed three basic means that people use to cope with this panic, as illustrated in Figure 3.

In Figure 3A, the large arrow going from right to left shows the individual's attempt to rid himself of the panic by directing the panic against others in the environment. Rick (p. 81) dem-

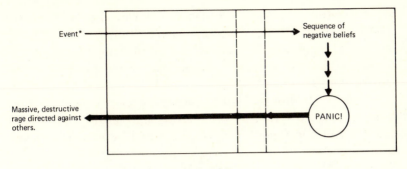

Figure 3A

onstrated this sequence in his overreaction to the taunting by the drunken man. Other examples will be shown in Chapter 7. This means of managing the panic is most frequently seen in people labeled as sociopathic individuals, explosive personalities, habitually assaultive individuals, and some manic patients and alcoholics.

In Figure 3B, the large arrow going from right to left shows the individual's attempt to rid himself of the panic and worthlessness by directing the self-punishing rage against himself. This behavior may take the form of an overdose, wrist slashing, accidents, acute paralyzing depression, brief psychotic episode, or a period of manic excitement. The actions are clearly self-punishing, usually brief, and relieving in quality. People who

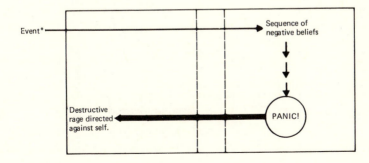

Figure 3B

behave in this fashion may be labeled as having primitive hysterical character, borderline personality disorder, cyclothymic personality, or masochistic character. Also included in this group are some manic–depressive patients and some severely obsessional patients.

Figure 3C shows a third mechanism of dealing with this sense of panic. Individuals who use this mechanism tend to contain the panic in rage-filled thoughts and fantasies. These fantasies are both repressed (forgotten) and suppressed (intentionally put aside but readily available to one's awareness). The desperation and rage are partially expressed in phobic concerns (unreasonable fears of situations or objects), or in psychosomatic illnesses. Some of the panic also appears in the individuals' chronic dissatisfaction and criticism of themselves and others. When the inner capacity to contain the panic fails and the phobic–critical–somatizing behavior no longer contains the panic, the individual may experience brief episodes of disorganizing anger, seemingly out of character. After the episode, the individual is humiliated and chagrined but does not understand the outburst. Such individuals have little perspective about the

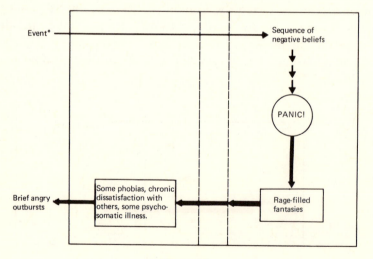

Figure 3C

origins of what occurred and cannot guard themselves against re-currences. They are frightened because their behavior seems to be out of their control.

For these people, control and appearance are important is-sues. They tend to be outwardly successful but derive no satis-faction from their accomplishments. Frequently, they report knowing the style and technique of human relationships but have no feeling for it. They experience life as a compulsively performed ritual. Except for occasional brief lapses, these indi-viduals tend to abuse alcohol and other drugs in a controlled manner. In the author's experience, these people use amphet-amines to accelerate their work performance as opposed to plea-sure seeking that has little personal meaning. Such people may have diagnoses of depressive character, phobic character, hys-terical personality, schizoid character, schizoid borderline per-sonality, or obsessional character.

Although there are other ways in which one might concep-tualize the foregoing material, I have attempted to present a more unified approach that has practical use for the beginning therapist. If one accepts it as a useful device rather than as a complete explanatory theory, it can be combined with other hy-pothetical constructs and approaches.

Some initial clarifications of this perspective are necessary. The individual with the alleged developmental defect (the sense of being nothing and its attendant panic) may use all three de-scribed means of dealing with the panic at various times in his life. At any particular time, one form will usually predominate over another. Some people may use the same mechanisms for days, months, or years before shifting. The more distressed the individual, the more rapid the shifting from one form of destruc-tiveness to another.

Use of drugs (alcohol and other chemicals), destructive be-havior, or compulsive work can be viewed as means of trying to contend with and contain the ongoing sense of worthlessness and panic. When the internal pressures increase, these faulty mechanisms fail and an explosion of feeling and behavior occurs (Figure 3).

The reader must keep in mind that what is presented here relates to the underlying predisposition to use impulsive behavior. Each means of behavior has its own inherent properties and problems that must be addressed in treatment along with the underlying concept. An active alcoholic, who is still drinking regularly, has impulse-control problems specifically relating to the chemical effect of alcohol. These effects must be addressed before any psychological therapy is useful. Similarly, the barbiturate addict in withdrawal, and for weeks afterward, is still responding to chemical and biological changes related to barbiturate use. The effects of the behavior or substance that is abused need consideration in the design of treatment. Although one may want to help the individual to comprehend and resolve the conflicts related to the sense of worthlessness, the *initial* stages of treatment must be different. The alcoholic may need detoxification, Alcoholics Anonymous, and a halfway house for months or years before some form of more insight-oriented therapy is useful. The impulsive borderline personality may need a brief custodial hospitalization and a period of reality-oriented psychotherapy before addressing the issues motivating the self-destructive behavior.

Several concepts do need clarification. Figure 1 shows two states in the individual: the external view (aware) and the internal view (partially aware). These do not correspond to the postulated states of consciousness and unconsciousness. The external view does involve a conscious awareness of how one views oneself in relation to one's environment, as well as some sense of the perspective others may have. This view is modified by one's automatic (unconscious) defenses. These automatic defenses are psychological maneuvers constructed by the individual, *without the individual's awareness*. They serve to protect the individual and to help him cope and adapt. When defenses become so cumbersome as to interfere with satisfying their function, they are designated as pathologic.

The internal view of oneself does not correspond exactly to the unconscious in ego psychology. The internal view is more akin to preconscious and moderately suppressed areas of awareness. Although an individual may deny the existence of an internal view, it is easily demonstrated and elicited into consciousness during therapy. The unconscious—while apparent in dreams, forgetting, slips of the tongue, automatic behavior, etc.—is less readily available to the approach of this text. The work described here moves from interpersonal awareness to intrapsychic awareness to the point of preconscious issues.

A schema that uses the constructs of ego psychology is more complicated (Figure 4) and less useful in this clinical work. The system shown in Figures 1, 2, and 3 can be used by the patient and the therapist in their work, as is shown in Chapter 7.

Much of the preceding material draws upon the premise that individuals have the capacity to observe their own thoughts, memories, feelings, impulses, and behavior. This correlates roughly to the observing ego in ego psychology. In discussions with colleagues, there is frequently a question as to the state of development of the observing ego in impulsive people. My experience with addicts and other impulsive people leads me to believe that they do have a self-observant capacity that does note thoughts, feeling, behavior, etc. This capacity can integrate these experiences and draw conclusions from the process. Yet, the understandings derived from this sequence are immobilized when the individual experiences the panic state.

> Bob, a polydrug abuser in therapy for 2 years, reported, "I know it's crazy. It makes no sense, but each time Sue turned to talk to someone else at the party, I felt explosive. She wasn't making a pass or really ignoring me. It was just normal conversation. I felt so enraged with her for not paying attention to me. Each time she turned back I felt relieved. Finally, I had to do something. I began gulping straight vodka." Bob became argumentative and passed out. His subsequent comments about that incident were: "I know what I want is impossible. No one can pay attention to you every minute of every day, but when I feel that way, no matter what I've decided or planned, I have to do something right away! I can't stop!" Bob is a highly skilled professional who uses the patterns outlined in Figures 3B and

3C. In spite of very clear understandings and experiences, his observations and resolve do not help him when he is confronted by his own sense of being worthless. His capacity to observe, correlate, integrate, and conclude seem to be present but powerless when the emotion is overwhelming.

Guilt and Conscience

Within the impulsive person, there exists a sense of guilt and a conscience roughly equivalent to the superego in ego psychology. The overt lack of remorse, guilt, or responsibility noted in some impulse-ridden people does not belie the existence of a sense of personal responsibility. While the individual may deny the experience of direct guilt, it appears in the self-punishing behavior and in the internal sense of being bad and reprehensible. In most instances, the development of a mature conscience has been distorted and halted. This unmodulated, primitive conscience frequently exists out of the patient's awareness (in the unconscious) and exacts a heavy price. Barbara (p. 46) demonstrated this quality. I have had contact with only a few individuals in whom it was difficult to find this personality aspect. These exceptions were cold, calculating individuals who were less prone to respond to provocation. Their outwardly destructive behavior, while vicious and deadly, was carried out with precision. Such precision is in marked contrast to the poorly planned, impulsive behavior one usually sees in addicted people. One of these individuals was a professional killer, another a highly educated medical professional. These people came close to fitting the description of the conscienceless psychopath. In my experience with impulsive people, such "psychopaths" are uncommon.

Figure 4 is a basic ego-psychology construct of personality functions. The enclosed area indicates the quantity of any particular aspect of the personality that is conscious, preconscious, or unconscious. Thus, according to this construct, the superego has

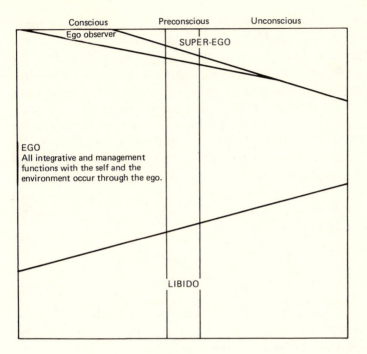

Figure 4

a much smaller representation in the conscious experience of the individual than in the unconscious experience.

Inadequate Personal Relationships

Loss and premature separation from needed adult nurturance deprive the individual of the opportunity to develop integrated concepts of people as composites of positive, negative, and neutral traits. The child tends to view people as "good" or "bad." The good are accepted completely, without question, and the bad are harshly rejected. This failure to have a more realistic, integrated picture of people accounts for part of the person's difficulty in forming lasting human relationships. Not only does the individual feel personally worthless, he is constantly viewing people as all good or all bad. He cannot see the presence of both qualities in the same person. It is incomprehensible. The constant change in relationships represents a searching out of the original lost, perfect parent. The individual perceives a fragmentary quality in the new acquaintance as representative of the whole lost parent. He is involved in a compulsive pursuit of the original lost person in order to resume the interrupted growth process. When the new "good" person demonstrates a negative trait, the individual rejects him as totally bad, unfulfilling, and deceiving. He reexperiences the initial loss and panics. When he runs out of energy and can no longer pursue the lost parent, drugs may temporarily allay the disappointment and depression.

Summary

In summary, impulsive behavior is a manifestation of an underlying ego defect. This defect is an inability to manage the emotional response to the belief that the individual is totally worthless and unlovable. The individual develops this defect when, between the ages of 3 and 7 years, there is a permanent loss of maternal nurturing care that had seemed potentially available. In many instances, it was only an illusion of adequate nurturance that was lost. At this time of change, there is no available and adequate substitute.

This change in maternal availability occurs when the child is struggling to develop internalized impulse control and self-esteem. The loss brings about the fixation of the early, poorly formed, and rigid conscience and is followed by panic, impulse-control problems, and self-punishment. These reactions are constantly replayed in present circumstances as the individual tries to deal with the initial loss.

This sequence usually reemerges in adolescence. This is the time when the individual is once again faced with the issues of growth, separation, impulse control, and personal responsibility. Because he is missing basic developmental experiences, he cannot progress beyond this repetitive cycle. The abuse of substances is an attempt to treat and relieve the distress.

The first four chapters provide a description of the author's theoretical and experiential perspectives. The following chapters present issues and techniques for the day-to-day use of these perspectives in clinical practice. Again, the work process is that of beginning with interactional awareness and moving toward intrapsychic understanding.

CHAPTER 5

Games

Introduction

Calling complex human interactions a game has a slick, insensitive quality. It fails to recognize the important, subtle issues that influence interactions. Such a simplification denies the multiple factors that enter into any personal negotiation and implies that there is only one important determining quality. It may also imply a judgment.

In spite of these drawbacks, the game concept is useful in communicating a number of views and is used here as a vehicle for that purpose. The games herein described show that both staff and patients may use the same techniques to deal with anxiety and the need for emotional discharge.

The game system also demonstrates that all of us may rationalize with words and intellect. Thus, our behavior may convey the very thought or feeling we wish to ignore. It is then clear why both staff and patients must learn to pay attention to their own inner responses and to deal with them. Failure to do this undermines treatment and leads to frustration and futility.

For these purposes, I have chosen to use the game model. It is useful only to sensitize one to the complexity of human interactions. The person seriously interested in understanding human behavior will have to go beyond this introduction.

After you have understood several games, you may find them repetitious. If you have gotten what you want from them, move on to Chapter 6 and return to the other examples later.

I have previously described games as situations in which there is a discrepancy between the overt or stated goal and the goal actually sought after.

Games can occur at three levels of consciousness. Some are consciously planned deceptions in which the perpetrator is fully aware of his deviousness. In others, the person initiating the game has a vague "feeling" of the true nature of his purpose: "I knew that it would work out that way, I had a feeling about it." "The thought occurred to me, but I didn't pay any mind." Thus, it occurs at a preconscious level of organization.

At the third level of consciousness, the gaming person is unaware of the discrepancy between his goals. These unconscious games represent automatic responses and repetitions of habitual situations. Frequently, they had started earlier in life as conscious games. After many repetitions, they have become automatic and unplanned responses to people and situations.

Underlying the conscious use of games is the belief that an indirect approach is the only way that will work. The person believes that openly moving toward an objective would mean certain failure: "If people knew what I really wanted, they would refuse me." The fact that the game is a personal statement of hopelessness is an issue of which the player must be made fully aware. His sense of inadequacy must be brought to consciousness and explored before resolution occurs. Staff members who find themselves gaming must also reach a similar understanding. Staff and patients both use the game style; the difference is usually one of degree, not motive.

A person with a self-destructive personality frequently is aware that the helper has both sadistic and aggressive impulses and is uncomfortable with them. The patient may use this knowledge to undermine treatment. Professional helpers frequently deny these impulses. They argue that they could not do their job if they felt anger and sadism. Yet, the choice of role as a helper frequently represents both a sublimation and a reaction against such feelings.

Persons in the medical professions frequently avoid the role of custodian and judge. They refuse to play the role of limit setter unless they are able to couch their actions in terms of being "in the patient's best interest." How many patients have received medication or electroshock therapy or have been committed to hospitals because of the physician's unacknowledged hostility?

Work with a neurotic patient may at times make the professional counselor bored, frustrated, or angry. Passive aggression may be mobilized in the helper. Rarely does the patient's emotional state require active intervention on the part of the counselor.

The psychotic patient initially makes his plight apparent. The counselor actively intervenes by offering comfort and structure to the painfully deluded, confused person. Later in treatment, the primitive, emotional material that emerges may cause the helper to become restive, frightened, bored, or angry. Such feelings may lead him to act inappropriately. Thus, the neurotic and the psychotic patient may arouse anxiety and defensiveness in the counselor.

The person with a self-destructive character disorder represents an immediate threat to the helper. Here is a person who doesn't acknowledge the need for help. Thus, he begins by denying the value of the counselor.

Frequently, a person with such character problems is facile with words and intellect and has no need for honesty. He uses the intellectual skills of the counselor but ignores the basic requirements of honesty. His characteristic mode of behavior becomes an assault upon the counselor's personal restraints.

The patient has no overt complaints and therefore removes the counselor's usual defensive maneuver of attributing maladaptive behavior to "sickness." Indeed, in many ways the patient seems normal. His self-destructive actions are usually accom-

panied by a life style that gives free reign to allegedly pleasure-
seeking impulses. There is a consistent history of self-
indulgence. Free of responsibility, the individual goes from
excess to excess, living an allegedly "high life." The uninitiated
counselor tends to see the patient as "normal" or like himself in
many ways because of verbal skill and lack of complaint. This
becomes frightening to the counselor because he "knows" that
there must be differences!

His identification with the patient leads the counselor to increasing anxiety about the restraints of his own conscience upon
his instinctual desires. The patient uses his awareness of the
helper's anxiety: "Haven't you ever been drunk or used pot? So
what's the difference between you and me?" He makes the neo-
phyte counselor feel that the temporary loosening of his superego restraints is equivalent to the patient's prolonged lack of
such restraints.

To the novice helper, a second threat emerges. Anxiety
about his own instinctual breakthrough leads to fantasies about
restraint of the patient. It is not unusual for the helper to
wonder if jail or a different hospital wouldn't be better. The
patient is a personal threat in that he has come to represent
the counselor's repressed impulses. The helper is in a bind: to
act upon his own responses out of defensive needs would be
inappropriate, yet the patient frequently demands stringent responses. *The sensitive counselor, uncomfortable about setting
limits, is not sure if he is objective about the needs of the patient
or is merely responding to his own inner defensiveness.* He is
aware that the patient sees him as the enforcer of society's demands, and he does not want to confirm this view. Because he is
unsure of himself, he becomes vulnerable to self-doubt when
the patient raises the specter of a nontherapeutic personal motivation as the cause for some restriction.

These are some of the factors that may have caused psychiatrists in general to avoid treating persons with destructive character disorders and may have led to the assumption that such
people are untreatable. It is no accident that prisons and the
chronic hospitals tend to be geographically isolated, fortresslike
enclosures. This need to isolate and hide individuals who pose a

threat to our own internal controls may have been instrumental in creating such institutions.

For the experienced counselor who has come to understand his own conflicts about aggression, sexuality, and sadism and has satisfactorily resolved them, treatment of patients with destructive character disorder has become possible and rewarding. The principles of dynamic psychotherapy are a valuable basis for planning treatment. Yet, it is easy to go wrong. The following examples of games between staff and patients testify to my own personal failures and those of other staff members as well as of patients. These same errors are repeated daily in other institutions. In the discussions of these games, I give both the staff's version and the patients' version where possible.

Kinds of Games

Killing with Kindness

This is a game in which the helper avoids dealing with a person's deviant behavior by taking the line, "I don't want to upset him," or "It seems to be such a drastic response. It is kinder to him not to deal with it." The real reason is that the counselor feels personal discomfort in clarifying the problem and feels that there is potential for serious consequences.

> *Staff's version:* Lee, 24, had transferred to the hospital directly from three years in the penitentiary. He was a thin, attractive man with an impish sense of humor and the ability to win people over. Several times during his stay in the Lexington center he violated rules of conduct: he disrupted meetings, possessed drugs, and failed to give certified urines for testing. By the established rules of the institution, he should have been expelled. Each time he was caught in a violation, he vehemently denied it and alleged that others were involved or that there were extenuating circumstances. When faced with incontrovertible evidence, he would plead not to be sent back to prison: "You people can't send me back." He would describe in woeful details the misery of prison life. Each time, the staff responded by

failing to adhere to the rules of conduct and gave Lee "another chance" to stay at the center.

When his escapades could no longer be ignored, he tearfully acknowledged all of his previous misdeeds and by a show of honesty won yet another opportunity to stay with the program. At no time, however, was he asked to demonstrate by consistent behavior and use of good judgment that he was committed to understanding and changing himself. He left the institution after the mandatory 6-month treatment period and was therefore no longer in danger of being returned to jail to serve out the rest of his sentence. Within 2 weeks of discharge, he was dead of a heroin overdose. Street reports had indicated that he had knowingly used "bad dope" from the day of discharge.

Had Lee been forced to live within the established regulations, he would certainly have been returned to prison. Admittedly, prisons have a miserable record of rehabilitation. However, this man had already survived 3 years in prison, and if returned there, he could have been available for future work. His behavior in the center made it evident that he was in no way altered and would most likely resume his self-destructive behavior. No one had effectively demanded that he change. His destructive behavior received tacit approval when he did not have to face the established consequences of his behavior. *Each successful manipulation of the staff reinforced his belief that his goal should be more skillful manipulation rather than personal change.*

The staff had kept themselves comfortable by avoiding their job. It was clear that Lee was demanding to be firmly dealt with and dropped from the program. Like a child, he tested the limits and found them weak. Yet the staff could not live with this concept because it would necessitate their involvement in his potential return to jail. They saw their own role in this decision as more significant than his behavior. It would have been appropriate for the staff to tell him that they would not send him to prison but that he would send himself as a result of his behavior. They were not compelling him to violate the rules, of which he knew the consequences. This episode occurred during the unit's early

formation and caused a significant reevaluation by the staff
of their own roles.

Killing with kindness does not always imply avoiding difficult decisions. Frequently it means ignoring an issue.

John was a 32-year-old male who portrayed himself as
a comfortable transvestite homosexual. He dressed in female clothing and spoke and acted in a caricature of seductive femininity. Neither staff nor patients questioned his
view of himself nor attempted to delve into his underlying
feelings. During a meeting, he stated repeatedly that he
was comfortable with his homosexuality. A review of his
past history and clinical behavior led the interviewer to
raise some questions regarding his early relationship with
his mother and his later pattern of self-destructive behavior.
These questions provoked the emergence of an outpouring
of anguish, rage, and depression. John began elaborating
previously unrelated material about his unhappiness and
loneliness. His dissatisfaction with himself and his antici-
pation of a bleak future became evident. There was ample
material to show that the unhappy loss of his manhood was
the price he paid to maintain his relationship with his
mother. The connections were apparent to him as he spoke.
As was true of other patients, he seemed glad to find someone who would not avoid talking about these painful issues.
Everyone was amazed at the depth of his unhappiness.

Following the conference, the staff reviewed its own
reluctance to deal with this man. They had been afraid to
upset him because he said that he was satisfied with himself. In reality, the frank discussion of homosexuality frightened them. To avoid their own discomfort, they had ignored John's behavior, which had amply demonstrated his
despair prior to the conference.

Patients' version: The tendency is to defend a person
whose behavior is clearly deviant. Even in situations in
which there is no danger of a patient's facing severe consequences, the other patients prefer to ignore, or to defend,
their fellow patient against the realistic evaluation of his behavior. This makes it easier for him to avoid seeing his own

role and facing its consequences. The result is continued self-destructive behavior. On the surface, the patients are banding together in a show of group loyalty. In reality, they are protecting themselves from the risk of future criticism. If they were to evaluate each other honestly, then no one would be safe from such scrutiny.

Thus, they perpetuate a situation in which no one is asked to alter himself. Since their previous behavior has been suicidal (use of drugs) and there is no change, they will most likely continue to be self-destructive and may kill themselves. Is it really a kindness to share your drugs with a friend? Yet, what could be more deadly than giving access to an unknown substance in a contaminated container when the consequences of such usage are physically and emotionally deadly.

Contracts

This is the street term that refers to a mutual agreement between individuals or groups to avoid acknowledging a situation or dealing with an issue. Contracts can be explicit or nonverbal.

Staff's version: During a staff group meeting, the discussion focused upon the negative and passive–aggressive attitude of one of the staff members. He was responding, when he paused, turned slightly, and smiled at the woman next to him. She returned his smile knowingly but said nothing. When she was asked about the interchange, she blandly replied, "Oh, it was nothing." Further comments made it clear that there was indeed something shared by the two of them but that she would not reveal it as "it had nothing to do with the group." A silence followed. The group's ongoing progress was interrupted because a contract of silence between two individuals had not been broken. Further progress could not be made. The man's attitude could not be better understood because he was refusing to divulge the hidden issue. His behavior was supported by his friend and colleague, who agreed not to share her ideas. Both would have criticized patients for doing the same thing in their group.

The staff and the patients can collaborate in a contract. The patients act "therapeutic" in groups and conduct "business as usual" outside of the group. The staff and the patients ignore this discrepancy, because they are more comfortable with the belief that their work is actually accomplishing its goal.

Peace at Any Price

This game is a variation on contracts. It is based upon none of the participants' wanting to expend more than the minimal amount of energy. Usually, a situation exists in which a decision is clear to all participants, who in order to avoid the consequences, predict dire results if the necessary action is taken.

The game of peace at any price goes on whenever a staff member or a patient fails to pursue an issue that needs to be explored. To do so would anger someone, so peace is gained by avoidance of the person's anger. The game is played out when unrealistic demands are met.

> *Staff's version, Example 1:* The central administration of the center at Lexington made a sudden policy decision regarding my treatment unit. The decision undermined the ongoing program. Staff members were both angry and hurt. They felt that further efforts to improve the program would run into equally disheartening results. The idea of openly discussing the issue with members of the administration was discarded as useless and likely to cause trouble, and administrative reprisal. Therefore, say nothing and gain "peace at any price."
>
> The development of the unit had been based upon the principle of open discussion of controversial issues. Yet, the general consensus in this instance was to avoid such a discussion for fear of reprisal. At the next meeting with the administration, the nuclear staff group brought up the issue for discussion. The administrator attempted to avoid the issue. On direct questioning, the administrator became angry, and a heated argument ensued. Although the specific policy was not altered, the unit's position in regard to

the hospital was clarified and strengthened. The unit director was given greater latitude in operating the unit's program. Within the staff, there was a greater feeling of internal unity coupled with some foreboding of administrative reprisal.

For several weeks, the administrator who had been present at the meeting showed his displeasure in critical comments, but none of the predicted reprisals occurred.

Had the issue been avoided, the principle of open discussion would have been lost, and the concept that "might makes right" would have been supported. The staff could not have wholeheartedly demanded openness from their patients when they themselves did not believe it could work. Anxiety and worry were the price paid for the greater sense of commitment to *proven* principles. Here peace at any price was avoided.

Example 2: One evening the doctor on call was summoned because a patient on another unit had been seen with a hatchet and large scissors after an argument with a fellow patient. Fearing violence, staff members did not attempt to deal with him directly, nor did they want the doctor on call to see the patient. Instead, they had another patient act as an intermediary.

Staff members, including the unit administrator, were paralyzed by their own fears of violence. At the direction of the unit administrator, the doctor was instructed to do nothing but wait until morning. (Yet, the patient could not be allowed to keep these weapons. They were a real danger to everyone in the environment.) Waiting and doing nothing would avert an immediate, violent confrontation, but all that would be gained was a fearful, transient peace at a horrible price. The doctor was extremely dissatisfied and informed the patient who was doing the negotiating that the armed man's behavior would be reported to senior administrators in the morning as a major violation of the institution's rules. The report would be submitted, no matter what the armed man did, and would be forwarded to Federal officials. If, however, he voluntarily turned over the weapons, that also would be included in the report.

Upon being informed that the decision to report the

man's actions was unequivocal and unalterable, the patient turned in both weapons within 5 minutes. This followed 2½ hours of fruitless negotiations.

This affair had many implications:

1. To discuss the surrender of weapons over a 2½-hour period supported the idea that there was something to negotiate. This is ridiculous!

2. Using another patient as a negotiator implied that his safety was less important than a staff member's. Though the patient was perhaps more easily antagonized by staff members, there was no guarantee that he would not turn upon a fellow patient. In fact, he first brandished the weapons after an argument with another patient.

3. *No treatment can be successful when the patient believes that his own violent impulses can control the situation. Peace at any price is really no peace. It is just an anxious truce that delays the making of the necessary decision and exacerbates the outcome.*

Secret Deals

This game might be called "I am your special friend." It is a variant of a contract game and may be played between a staff member and a patient. The patient shares information with a staff member on the condition that the information will be kept private and will result in no action. Thus, an open exploration of the issue and a resolution are precluded. When the game is played behaviorally, the staff member meets the patient's demands, spoken or implied, without questioning the appropriateness of such actions.

When the game is played among patients, they usually agree to keep specific shared information secret. In reality, the person who acts as the friend and collaborator is only promoting self-destructive activity by failing to bring it out into the open for examination.

Patients frequently make use of secret agreements with other patients or staff members in order to obtain relief from burdensome conflicts. They react as if the confidant, once he knows the issue, has taken the burden of responsibility for the patient. This is seen dramatically in psychiatric hospitals when one patient tells another of a suicide plan but binds the confidant to secrecy. The friendship agreement binds the recipient of such information not to question the decision to commit suicide and, in addition, not to reveal it. The recipient frequently becomes upset as he wrestles with his dilemma: whether to tell someone and risk his friend's rage or to be silent and allow the friend to kill himself. At the same time, the individual who has shared the information has a sense of comfort as his confidant struggles with the impossible choice.

Staff's version, Example 1: One day a nurse's aide approached a unit physician. She had secret information, but before revealing it, she wanted to know exactly what would be done. The doctor responded that he could not guarantee his response without knowing the nature of the information. He asked her to trust their mutual ability to reach a reasonable understanding. She resisted. He pointed out that by entering a conspiracy in which she shared information with the patients but could not confer with other staff, she prevented herself from obtaining the consultation she felt she now needed. The result was that the patient was being denied necessary assistance. A program for mutual consultation was being undermined.

She responded by wryly smiling and saying, "Oh, don't worry, I've got my ways of getting information." She was asked how she used such information. With reluctance, she acknowledged that its use was limited. As she was usually pessimistic about being effective in her job, it made her feel important. The usefulness of this shared information to the patient was next to nothing. The covert goal of her game was to increase her sense of effectiveness. She was treating herself at the patient's expense.

Example 2: A variation of this game is to comply with demands in order to avoid anxiety. One evening when on call for the center in Lexington, a doctor was summoned to the women's unit to see a patient who had superficially cut her wrist. She had done this numerous times in the past.

When he arrived, the nurse was holding the patient's hands
and rocking her gently, saying soothing words as one would
to a frightened child. The patient seemed calm and somewhat disdainful. While the doctor was preparing to suture
the patient's wrist, the nurse anxiously ran to get water and
cigarettes for the patient. While suturing, the doctor spoke
to the patient about the episode and asked whether further
self-injury was probable that night. Before she could answer, the nurse repeatedly stated that she was sure that
there would be no further episodes. She made these statements pleadingly. Later, in private, the patient casually dismissed the nurse's behavior as evidence of anxiety: "Oh,
she's just scared."

The nurse had busied herself in ostensibly calming the
patient but was actually meeting her own needs. There was
no discussion, however, of the patient's internal distress or
her primitive way of calling for help by cutting herself. The
nurse had said, "Oh, I didn't ask her why. I didn't want to
know about all that." Instead, her efforts were directed
toward satisfying the patient's every wish in the hopes of
forestalling further disruptive episodes.

There are many implications in this response. It gave
the patient immediate gratification and reinforced her use
of self-injury as a means of gathering attention and concern.
It failed to deal with the motivation for such behavior. The
staff member's anxious response conveyed the message, "I
will do anything that you want, but please don't upset me."
With the focus thus shifted to the staff member's anxiety,
the patient had a means of further manipulation.

Distractions

In this game one issue is used to cloud another.

    Staff's version: A staff member who played a significant
role in the unit at Lexington made a habit of avoiding staff
meetings. Although he demanded a say in the structure of
the unit, he found the meetings too demanding. After
attending several, he stopped.

    When asked to attend the meetings in order to take

part in policy decisions, he responded with an effort to distract attention from the major issue. Unable to discuss the emotional demands that these meetings made on him, he described the meetings as boring and a waste of time. It was clear that the major issue for him, however, was the intense conflict he felt about discussing the reasons for his actions. He did not want to explain them. When he did attend, people questioned his reasons for decisions. Frequently, he became furious at being questioned and would leave the meeting for other business. The meetings were too demanding. He was attempting to avoid the real issue of personal discomfort.

Patients' version: A patient was denied a privilege that he was convinced he was entitled to receive. He told a staff member that as a consequence he would burn the United States flag. When staff members reacted to this threat by talking about flag burning, he responded that the government and society had failed him. The staff rose to the bait and began defending United States policy and culture. The patient had successfully distracted the staff from discussing whether he was entitled to receive something that he in fact had not earned.

The staff did not discuss the lack of logic in his response. What did burning the flag have to do with his demand to have an unearned pass? They had fallen into his trap of discussing American society.

"I'm No Racist"

This is a subdivision of the distraction game. Racism is evident in all institutions—in both overt and more subtle forms. Because such prejudices represent learned responses that interfere with reasonable interactions, they need to be examined as they appear. At times, however, they are used to cloud a realistic appraisal of other issues. An individual may label an issue "racial" as a way of avoiding other more important issues.

Staff's version: Two men in a group requested a pass. One was black, one white. The white patient had clearly qualified by the institutional standards of behavior. The black man had not met the standards but implied that he would be denied the pass because of his race. The therapist recognized the ploy but decided to avoid the hassle and give them both passes. He thus undermined the working principles of the unit: "Oh Christ, they would have said I was prejudiced, and I didn't want to go through that again."

Obviously, the therapist allowed himself to be manipulated. He avoided the difficult task of distinguishing racism as a ploy from racism as a reality. The other patients understood the ploy and later stated that they knew the black man had not earned a pass. They had not spoken up earlier because they enjoyed the therapist's discomfort and enjoyed seeing a cohort "beat the system."

Poor Communication

Any number of individuals or groups can participate in this game. A plan is discussed and responsibility allocated. The issue is either poorly defined or poorly understood. As a result the plan fails through confusion. Several groups may then gain a negative advantage.

Staff–patients' version: During a holiday, two patients restricted from social activities because of drug use were informed that they were also forbidden to see the holiday movie. The patients, realizing that frequently there was confusion about such plans between different hospital shifts, sought out various staff members and asked permission to attend the movie. The nurses and aides repeated that they could not go. A physician was approached and questioned. He did not know of the agreement. Instead of asking the staff on the unit, he telephoned a senior staff person at home. The senior staff person had forgotten the agreement and allowed the restricted men to go to the movies.

The nurses and aides said nothing at the time. After several days of sullen behavior by these people, they asked, "What is the use of our doing a job, if we don't get support?" Finally, the situation was discussed. Superficially, it seemed to be the kind of error that is common in large institutions with many staff members. Overtly, it was a simple misunderstanding. All parties could deny responsibility. The nursing staff did not confront the physician and ask him to reverse himself. They were content to assume that they were misunderstood and oppressed. It was the easier way. They could rationalize their further conservation of effort by saying, "It's no use—we don't count anyway."

For his part, the physician could not admit that he was uninformed because he had been absent from the meetings. He felt that he had discharged his obligation by calling a senior man. His failure to consult with available staff did indicate his lack of respect for the knowledge or judgment of the subordinate staff. His devaluation of the subordinate working staff was clear. The senior staff man, home on holiday, made a hurried decision without refreshing his memory by calling the staff on duty. The patients received the immediate gratification of successful manipulation. This reinforced their attitude that deception is the most successful form of goal achievement.

Goal Disharmony

In this "game of games," two individuals or two groups agree upon the formulation of plans and guidelines. Neither side discusses the obvious fact that they do not share the same basic goal.

> *Staff–patients' version:* In establishing the unit, the staff formulated rules regarding the use of drugs in the institution: "An individual *might* be asked to leave the center if he was found to have used drugs once or twice. He would definitely be asked to leave if it was found that he had used drugs three times."
>
> In practice, no one was asked to leave before he had used drugs three times. The staff believed that a person might be serious in wanting treatment and yet might experience moments of despair or anxiety and give in to the desire to use drugs. The staff's premise was that the patients genuinely desired to stop using drugs.

In practice, the patients interpreted the rules as license for "two free shots" of drugs. They felt that they had the right to two episodes of drug use without fear of sanction. Thus, the rule, at least in the way it was enforced, promoted the use of drugs. The patients helped to write the guidelines but with the goal of being able to use drugs with minimal consequences. Their goal was different from the staff's, yet both agreed upon the initial guidelines.

Further evidence of separate goals was shown in another practice. The rules stated that a man could reveal institutional drug use within his group therapy setting without being subjected to institutional discipline. The hope was to explore and understand the motivation for drug use. If the patient gave no evidence of change after repeated confessions, he would be informed that he would no longer be immune from consequences.

In spite of this leniency, those found using drugs via random urine tests had uniformly failed to discuss drug use within their groups. It was clear that a rule based upon so-called reasonable expectations was not realistic in this situation because it failed to deal with a basic discrepancy. The groups did not share the same goal: drug abstinence and the understanding of personal motivation.

A more reasonable harmony was reached when the staff agreed that there was no compelling need to use drugs *within the institution.* They also noted that there was no evidence that the men shared with the staff the goal of abstinence. Consequently, three changes were made.

1. Any use of drugs not previously dealt with in group therapy became grounds for immediate dismissal from the program. This resulted in a significant drop in the use of opiates and barbiturates within the unit.

2. There was an increase in group therapy evaluation of individual instances of drug use within the unit, including marijuana.

3. Patients were no longer pushed into giving false reasons for entering the institution, namely, that they wished to overcome drug and character problems. They could freely acknowledge their actual reasons for entering the center without fearing rejection from the program.

They could openly state that their only motivation was to avoid prison sentences or to satisfy family pressure.

The true reasons for entry into the program eliminated one area of deception. Few addicts are motivated to character change; however, there was hope that once involved in the center's activities, they might begin to reevaluate themselves during the 6 months of treatment.

"Uh, Huh, I Knew It All Along"

In this game, an individual lives up to a poor expectation ("I knew you were bad") and thereby satisfies a second person. As soon as the negative expectation is met, the second person loses all interest; he is satisfied that he has been right. The offender becomes more alienated because he perceives that the "helper" is satisfied to see him only in negative terms. usually, the offender will not try to understand his own behavior.

> *Staff's version:* I was caught in this game when I suspected that a patient had returned from a leave with drugs. When his urine test showed positive for opiates and he actually dropped a packet of drugs out of his pocket, I experienced a sense of satisfaction. He was hopeless. The man had always seemed particularly obnoxious.
>
> Several days later, however, I realized that the patient had antagonized me by actively trying to disrupt and undermine the development of the program. Aware of this, I spoke to the man and learned that his attempt at disruption was related to his hatred of all authority and stemmed from early and current dealings with his father.
>
> Unfortunately, I had not seen this underlying issue sooner and had missed an opportunity to work with this man. I had confirmed my initial belief that the man was an obnoxious individual who could be dismissed along with his bothersome questions.
>
> *Patients' version, Example 1:* Several patients had worked with staff members early in the program in an attempt to change the attitude of their fellow patients. For their efforts, they were ostracized by their peers when they failed.

They became depressed and broke the rules of conduct as a way of doing penance and reentering their peer group.

The peer group then exacted even more severe penalties and showed none of their usual interest in helping these men avoid the consequences of their behavior. They made comments to these men about their "high and mighty" attitudes. The other patients had "always known they were no different," they said. They were happy once again to have proved that no addict can change. This relieved the pressure on the others to attempt change.

Example 2: There may be situations in which negative expectations are useful. In the center in Lexington, there were five men with whom numerous genuine efforts to change seriously self-destructive behavior were fruitless. It became evident that these patients were either persisting in drug use within the hospital or were planning to use drugs immediately upon release and were suicidal. However, they insisted that in spite of the evidence, they were not going to use drugs.

During an open meeting, I purposely presented the evidence of impending self-destructive behavior in a direct but moderately sarcastic manner. The five persons responded to this and saw the issue as a personal struggle between themselves and me. They said they would rather do anything than give me the satisfaction of being right. All five subsequently sent messages to the hospital via friends or mail, reassuring the staff that "for once he was wrong." The man who had been most suicidal figured out my ploy and discussed it with me upon readmission: "You were right about everything else, but I wouldn't give you the satisfaction of killing myself." Two of the others did return to drug abuse after several months of abstinence.

I do not intend to present this technique as a preferred one. It was a desperation maneuver that only temporarily succeeded. In spite of the fact that the somewhat sarcastic discussion was based upon a realistic appraisal of information, the gaming approach makes it a form of deception. While it is useful to present a realistic appraisal of a situation in a neutral manner, the introduction of sarcasm as a means of personalizing the discussion is a dangerous ploy.

The individual can believe that you really do wish him ill and believe him to be bad.

Sliding by, or "I'm No Trouble"

Patients and staff who play this game quietly comply with all demands placed on them. They are "invisible men," avoiding notice and scrutiny. Their active participation is minimal, despite their overt compliance. As patients they tend to win praise from untrained staff because they do nothing disruptive, and they receive support for their passivity. Although they do what is required, their attitude precludes any real growth.

Staff's version: The staff person who slides by usually fulfills the role of a "good guy." He jokes with patients and supports the feeling that "we're all just friends." He is usually quiet in staff meetings and openly supports the majority on any issue. He does not contribute new ideas or his own point of view; in fact, he does not involve himself in any way. His disinterest is sensed by the patients, and his failure to participate makes a greater burden for those who must pull his weight. The patients use his lack of involvement in rationalizing their own lack of participation: "If he isn't interested, why should I be?" When questioned, such a person will defensively retreat to a recitation of the rules covering his job or will state that he only does what he is asked to do.

Superficially, the invisible man is doing his share according to the rules. Beneath the surface, such individuals think change only leads to a worsening of the situation. They share the same beliefs as the patients.

Patients' version: Carl, a 35-year-old, robust individual, worked more than 50 hours per week although he was only required to work 20. He was a polite, model patient. His isolated job removed him from observation. When he was requested to work only 20 hours and remain on the unit, he admitted that he felt great discomfort in talking with people and in dealing with his own anger. He could not tolerate discord and in spite of his great size and strength feared anyone who spoke harshly. Constant pressure led to his admission that he feared criticism from his aged father and anyone else who indicated displeasure with him. If he had been allowed to "slide by," he would never have begun to deal with this crippling characteristic. He had previously used drugs to blot out the anxiety related to experiencing rage and dealing with his father.

Good Guy–Bad Guy, or Splitting

In this game, the person deals with internal conflicts by assigning parts of these conflicts to different persons in his environment. He sits on the sidelines while others struggle with his issues. Their struggle temporarily relieves him of pain but does not resolve his situation.

Staff–patients' version, Example 1: In one therapy group, two co-therapists had markedly different views of how to work with impulse-ridden people. One therapist wanted to follow a rigorous line, with rewards for behavior he considered appropriate. He seemed to view the group members as different from himself and called them lazy, immoral "jerks" who couldn't change. The other therapist wanted to make no demands and be totally flexible. In an idealistic way, he felt that all people were good and that a warm, open approach would win everybody over to his beliefs in the basic goodness of men. Although the two therapists talked about their differences, neither could listen and no resolution occurred. Their apparent differences were furthered by the group. Seeing the differences in style and perspective at the outset, the group began ostracizing and criticizing the more demanding therapist, while praising and supporting the more flexible therapist.

The more demanding and punitive therapist withdrew and became a nonparticipant. This continued for a brief time, until it was found that four of the nine group members were consistently using drugs. The group's internal conflict between its rigid, puritanical father and its indulgent father was not resolved. The role of the more rigorous therapist emerged when the group made it clear that they needed strict demands yet resented the imposition of these demands by others. Here the therapists' failure to resolve their differences (split) played into a destructive acting-out by the group.

In psychiatric hospitals dealing with impulsive people, it is common for some staff members to view a patient as warm, concerned, and giving, while others view the same person as angry, cold, provocative, and indifferent. Conflicts then occur among the staff over who has made the more correct observation. While the staff is in conflict, the patient is usually escalating his self-destructive behavior.

Further evaluation usually leads to the conclusion that both perspectives have some validity. The individual patient has presented a different facet of his personality to different members of the staff. When staff members fail to consider that they may be correctly viewing different parts of the individual's personality, they are unable to reach a resolution. Such a resolution is necessary if the patient is to be dealt with in a consistent manner that takes into account the conflicting aspects of his personality.

> *Example 2:* Leif was asked why he had such a hostile attitude toward a nurse with whom he had had little personal experience. He explained, "I could tell by the way she looked the first time I saw her that she would be a bitch. I know that type." He used subsequent selected observations to support this initial belief. When evidence to the contrary was brought to his attention, he saw it as an attempt to fool him. It was pointed out that his initial angry and provocative reaction to the nurse might have been a factor in causing the nurse to appear bitchy and controlling to him. His reply was, "She's a nurse; she is supposed to know how to act." He used as evidence his warm feelings for another nurse, whose slow speech and casual mode of dress told him that she was a good person. She also viewed him in positive terms.
>
> Subsequent discussion revealed that he believed that the more casually attired nurse must be sloppy and disdain-

ful of her physical self, as he was of himself. His internal conflict between the part of him that was more demanding on himself and the part that wished to be casual and sloppy had been displaced onto the persons of the two nurses. Fortunately, the nurses discussed their opposite appraisals of his character and confronted him with it. If they had not done this, each could have justifiably thought that her own observations were more accurate, and there would have been no discussion of the patient's inner conflict.

Patients' version: A patient who had appeared to be well on his way to a productive life during a previous admission was recommitted and appeared very depressed. He was an intelligent man who had been a convincing speaker. A physician who had seem him on the previous admission was struck by the alteration in his physical state. The patient sought out the physician and persuaded him to provide a methadone maintenance program. The physician agreed to this without consulting the staff members who were working with the man.

Several weeks later, at a staff conference, the split between the physician and the rest of the staff became apparent. Several staff members protested that all indications showed the man to be unreliable in a methadone program. After a period of argument in which the patient did not participate, the physician was convinced that indeed this was the case. When the patient learned that the physician and the staff were now discussing and resolving their differences, he became furious and impulsively left the hospital. During his third admission, he discussed the split in terms of his special relationship with the "good guy" doctor. He viewed this physician as a powerful individual who should have been able to overcome any staff opposition. He had counted on this and had put all of his efforts into winning this doctor's support while showing unreliable behavior to the rest of the staff. The other staff members, who had raised realistic questions, were "bad guys" because they would not go along with the plan.

While allowing this split to develop, the staff was unable to deal with the patient's poor planning and character deficiencies. Having initially won over the physician, he had placed all of his interest in obtaining methadone. His belief in the physician's omnipotence was supported by the fact that the doctor worked in isolation from the other staff members and therefore didn't know of their observations until the conference.

The patient, unable to resolve his own conflict between chronic methadone dependence and a difficult drug-free life, sought powerful allies outside of himself who would settle the issue for him. It is apparent that for this kind of splitting to occur, the staff must actively comply.

Jailhouse Lawyer

This is the game of finding legalistic loopholes that allow a person to avoid facing the origins or consequences of his behavior. The goal is to avoid facing a major issue by focusing on a lesser issue and wearing everyone out. Success occurs when everyone gives up and discards the issue as too complex or energy-consuming. Frequently, there is agreement to make a new rule that will cover the exact situation. *One cannot make rules to cover every situation and must depend upon reasonable expectations derived from shared objectives.*

Overtly, the person who is acting as a lawyer is seeking to protect his own or his pseudoclient's legal right. The fact that the setting in which this takes place is clinical, not legal, means little to him. *The focus is not upon the patient's behavior and its motivation but upon the legalistic discussion.*

> *Patients' version:* A patient was found acting suspiciously in the men's room. He was concealing a bottle of wine. Several feet away, there were two more bottles of wine under some towels. When asked for an explanation, he denied any knowledge of the bottles. Later, he stated that he thought they were soda bottles. Before further discussion could take place, a friend (jailhouse lawyer) stated that no one had actually seen the man with the bottles in his hands and that anyway it was quite possible that he really thought the bottles were soda. The fact that the man's

suspicious behavior had called attention to him was ignored.

To accept the "jailhouse lawyer's" argument would be
to fall into the trap of helping individuals avoid dealing with
their own behavior. Later, the patient acknowledged that
he knew the content of the bottles and had just bought
them. Several staff members, however, had been stymied
by the fact that there were no witnesses to the conceal-
ment. Nor could they discount the possibility (highly un-
likely) that he mistook a bottle of wine for a bottle of soda.
To fall into such deception invites repetition. The helper
needs to be comfortable in confronting a deception and
labeling it as such. If he does this angrily, however, or uses
it as a general characterization of the person ("You are a
complete liar"), then the value of the interaction is lost. The
clinical issue that arises in the context of dealing with the
behavior relates to understanding why the person decided
to act as he did. What were his choices, motivations, or options? How did he weigh the risks and benefits?

As in any system, there must be concern that a person
be given the benefit of the doubt. This leniencey should not
be stretched, however, to the ludicrous point where the
rules are used to condone obvious deception. This kind of
reverse logic is seen in the national advertising campaign
urging people not to help a good boy become bad by leaving
keys in a car. It is clear that keys in an ignition are an invitation to theft. It is also clear that "joyriding" can be a
minor legal offense. The overriding issue, however, is the
fact that the person stealing the car knows that he is stealing
and has *chosen* to do so. The advertising campaign implies
that the sight of keys in an ignition presents an irresistible
compulsion over which the individual has no control. Such
a point of view promotes irresponsibility: "I couldn't help
it."

One patient explained his theft of a tape recorder as
being the owner's fault because the owner did not have it
securely bolted to the cabinet. Another man explained his
shooting of a robbery victim as the victim's fault: "He made
it happen. It was his fault. He saw I had a gun. He
shouldn't have come at me."

The Lame Game

The player of the lame game presents himself as incapable of guile. He promotes the idea that he, "the lame," is too stupid to be deceptive. In the street, the addict uses this to win another individual's confidence. The target individual then feels safe and superior to the lame. He believes that he could not be deceived by this individual. Subsequently, the lame sells his item (dope, television, women) at what appears to be a very low cost. The target individual does not suspect that he is being duped because he has become overconfident.

In the institution, the patient may assume a lame role intellectually, emotionally, or physically. It can be a conscious and planned game or one that is automatic and habitual. The goal is to avoid a particular task or responsibility.

> *Patients' version, Example 1:* Clem was a man in his mid 50s with a 30-year history of intermittent polydrug use. During his staffing conference, he repeatedly stated that he was confused or that he misunderstood the issues being discussed. Slouching in his chair, he appeared somewhat bewildered and lacking in energy. He attributed this seeming inability to participate in a discussion to his age and lack of education as compared to that of the "skilled" physician. He drew attention to the fact that he was just a poor, uneducated man from the hills while the doctor came from a big city and had attended large universities.
>
> He was then asked how he had supported his family and his drug habit. For 30 years, he had avoided serious entanglement with the law and had adequately provided for the financial needs of both drugs and family—a considerable task. The man became hesitant, and the social worker gradually drew from him a history of successful gambling and confidence games. When asked how a person who seemed to be so intellectually slow could be a successful gambler and confidence man (support a family and drug habit while avoiding the law), the patient smiled, laughed, sat up, and said, "Well I guess you got me." As the confer-

ence continued, the patient spoke in a clear and energetic fashion. He characterized his previous attitude as one of his means of "getting by."

Example 2: During orientation meetings, Burt was repeatedly observed staring into space and playing with his hands. His answers to questions were mere grunts. He appeared to be retarded or psychotic.

During one of the meetings, however, another patient made a comment and Burt darted a quick glance at him in an angry and alert manner. He then resumed his dull, withdrawn stance. Questions were then raised as to whether these two men had any prior association outside of the institution. The man who had made the comment acknowledged that this was the case. He was then asked whether Burt had always appeared withdrawn and isolated. What was he like in the street? At first, the other patient was reticent, then he burst out laughing: "Man, Burt is laming you!" After swearing at his friend, Burt began speaking clearly and coherently and with no apparent deficiency or thought disorder. His appearance of retardation immediately disappeared.

Example 3: Gerry was an example of the automatic lame. He was a young man who constantly chattered and involved himself in the group's activities. He was quite accurate in pointing out other people's indiscretions or illogical comments. Whenever the group focused on him, he automatically cupped his hand to one of his ears as if he could not hear, or he claimed to misunderstand the idea. This went on for weeks until group members pointed it out to him. This selective hearing deficiency did not have any organic basis but was an automatic and unplanned response to uncomfortable material. He found he could avoid discomfort through these small maneuvers.

Forget the Past

This game is used regularly by persons suffering from character problems. In my experience, it has been generally used more by patients than by staff. Because their past record of achievement has been poor, such persons avoid taking into account past situations when planning current or future activities. They cannot learn from past situations, because they are compelled to maintain the perspective that they did not make mistakes—they were merely the victims of external forces and fate. Similarities between current and past situations are avoided because the individual believes that the future will only bring failure. He meets attempts to promote such a review with comments like, "Why bring that up? That was last week." Overtly, he is saying, "Do not judge me by my past behavior; that would be unfair to me." Covertly, the message is, "I cannot review the past because I see no evidence of change within myself." For change to occur there must be an uncritical but realistic review of similarities in previous situations. Where growth has occurred, it should be noted and supported. Where no growth has occurred, this should be noted and explored. From this, realistic planning can begin. Usually, the individual does not realize that *a major problem is his/her decision-making capacity. The process of taking in data, reviewing it, weighing options and outcomes, setting priorities, etc.—all of this is foreign.* When confronted with having to make decisions, these individuals become anxious about the outcome. *Having no belief or experience in successful decision-making, they relieve their anxiety by using familiar (reflexlike) decision patterns.* Thus, they make an automatic decision, even if they know it will have a poor result. They have a decision; they do not have to live with the anxiety and uncertainty of indecision. Thus, any decision, even a poor one, is less stressful than uncertainty. Reviewing the past and relating the similarity to the present raises self-doubts and anxiety in the individual.

In a treatment setting, the helper is obligated to show the similarities between past and present circumstances and to help the individual to review plans and thinking. At the same time, he should endeavor to help the individual to delay putting them into effect until the patient is more assured of a reasonable outcome.

Sulk

The person playing this game feels that he is being threatened but has no logical response other than to acknowledge his
own error. Because acknowledging the error is too painful, he
withdraws into a sullen, quiet position. In either action or
words, he says, "I don't want to talk about it or look at it anymore. I will deprive you of my involvement and you need me
more than I need you. See how you're upsetting me."

The sulk has two goals: (1) it may engender sympathy from
the people about him, who do not want to cause further discomfort; and (2) it carries an implied threat: "If you talk to me in this
way, I will not respond to you. I will not participate with you. If
you want me to be involved with you, you must not make me
look at myself." He invites a contract of mutual agreement to
avoid evaluation of some problem.

> *Staff's version:* Following a heated staff meeting in
> which several members criticized others for reneging on a
> particular commitment, some of those who were criticized
> said, "We won't discuss it if that's the way you feel!" We're
> just not going to do anything." In effect they were saying
> that their behavior should not be observed or discussed:
> "We should all comply and be pleasant, but we must not
> realistically appraise our situation."
> *Patients' version:* A patient violated a principle of the
> institution by hitting another person. The members of his
> group attempted to overlook the issue in order to help him
> avoid dismissal. When the therapist pointed this out and
> stated that the patient must examine his behavior and deal
> with it, one of the group members said, "You have had it
> easy so far, Dr. J. We have been very cooperative. But if
> you go on like that, we are not going to do anything about
> therapy. We'll just sit here." They would sulk. The possibil-
> ity that they could gain by working in therapy was dis-
> carded in the retreat to an infantile position. Sulking im-
> plied that the process of therapy was more for the benefit of
> the staff than to patients. As the group members made

clear, they were not participating in the group for themselves but were merely placating their therapist, who, in
fact, had been interested in their feigned goodwill.

Stir Him Up

Frequently, a staff member or a patient becomes involved
in a situation in which he has strong convictions. Other persons
note the level of personal interest and decide to play him along
in order to aggravate him. They have little interest in the issue
itself. Their only goal is to promote greater frustration on the
part of the interested party.

> *Staff–patients' version:* One day, two officials of the pa-
> tients' government had not shown up for a meeting that
> they were obligated to attend. A staff member who had in-
> vested a good deal of time and effort in the government said
> with concern and anger showing on her face, "Why weren't
> you there? You know you were supposed to be there; this is
> part of your job."
> As she became more and more animated, the two men
> lounged further back in their seats with looks of boredom
> on their faces. When she finished her statement with the
> question "Why?" one man yawned apathetically, "Gee, I
> didn't realize I was supposed to be there." The other one
> said, lazily, "Oh, I forgot; I think I fell asleep." Both of
> these remarks were contrived to exasperate her. After she
> left the room, they burst out laughing. The patients had
> purposely added insult to injury by denying any responsi-
> bility and failing to match the staff member's interest. Their
> exaggerated lack of concern was a further provocation. As in
> the sulk game, a basic position is that the other person has
> more to gain or lose by one's participation. *It is a reversal of
> interests.* Had the staff member confronted the individuals
> with less of a demonstration of personal investment, she
> might have accomplished more. The staff person was ex-
> pending the energy, not the patients. (See Game 8, goal
> disharmony.)
> We see this anytime two persons do not have equal in-

terest in an issue. As the helper becomes more active, the
patient becomes more passive. Addicts continually tell us of
parents, friends, clergymen, and other interested people
who spend great amounts of time, talking and exerting
themselves in the hope of convincing the individual to alter
his behavior. The more energy these other people expend,
the less interested the addict seems. *Whenever there is evidence that the helper has greater investment than the person seeking help, no useful results occur.*

Confrontation Avoidance

Most staff members and almost all patients avoid talking
with each other about deficiencies in behavior or attitude. Many
reasons are given for this: "They become so hostile." "He won't
listen; it's no use." The most frequently used reasons boil down
to three, which can be summarized as follows: (1) "The other
person will be hostile and will make me uncomfortable"; (2) "It
is cruel for me to hurt him by calling it to his attention; he already feels bad"; and (3) "He might notice some similar deficiency of mine."

There is, however, a more significant reason to avoid confronting an individual. For a staff member to confront a patient
effectively, he must give up his role and approach the patient
on a person-to-person level. *He must be able to show that a particular behavior or attitude represents poor judgment in terms
of the patient's own frame of reference.* It is foolish to appeal to
someone's sense of fairness, morality, responsibility, etc., when
his daily behavior gives repeated evidence that he holds a different standard than the observer. Staff members are unsure as
to their grounds in this situation. They cannot easily give up the
security of being right by virtue of their status or personal moral
belief. It is difficult to put oneself into someone else's frame of
reference and to prove that he is in error by his own standards.

The concept of confrontation has come to be identified with
a vigorous, verbal assault that leaves a person shorn of his necessary defenses. If, in fact, this is the nature of confrontation, it is
dangerous and destructive and must be avoided. A person must

never be shamed, humiliated, or degraded. The most effective confrontation that I have seen occurs when a person's situation is clarified quietly and directly. The confronting individual must convey that his interest is not in proving the other person wrong. He must make it evident that his only concern is in obtaining a more objective understanding of the individual and the motivation for his behavior. Beyond that, there is the interest in finding the source of his internal discomfort and devising a more satisfactory solution.

With this attitude, it has been possible to point out openly that a man is lying without causing him to respond with an excessively angry defense. By avoiding the "Ah ha, I've got you now" game, we focus upon the *underlying need to misrepresent facts* rather than upon the fact of lying itself. By doing this, we encourage the men to look at themselves with less fear of finding themselves deficient. The helper needs to understand that no one can tolerate being stripped of defenses and abandoned. All of us need defenses to keep functioning as best we can. *The goal is to help the patient see that he can safely give up maladaptive defenses because he has strengths and abilities that he was not aware of.* It is possible to do this in the context of a relationship in which one person can count upon the other to be honest, realistic, and nonpunitive.

For example, the need to lie is frequently rooted in a sense of personal deficiency. By exploring the specific deficiency in a noncritical way, the patient may learn that his supposed deficiency is nonexistent or less important than he previously believed. Where the deficiency does exist, exploration frequently reveals that it is alterable.

Focus on the Specific to Avoid the General Issue

When faced with an undesirable attitude or character trait, a person may attempt to avoid or discredit the problem by finding some minor discrepancy. He then focuses upon this discrepancy. This game clearly includes elements of avoidance and all-or-none behavior.

Patients' version: A patient was confronted with the fact that although he was the community leader, he missed meetings, slept while others worked, and claimed credit for work time when he was supposed to be at meetings. His sense of duplicity, entitlement, and laziness were the focal issues.

In defense, the patient chose to argue that *some* of the work time was valid. He avoided discussing his general lack of commitment (a chronic character problem that had been noted from early childhood). He acted as if proving that some of the work time was valid would totally discount the problem of his persistent past behavior. He acted as if finding one discrepancy absolved him from any requirement to observe his own behavior further.

A Rose by Any Other Name

In many treatment settings, patients are referred to by names that indicate that they are not patients, prisoners, addicts, etc. In Lexington, they were called residents. The reason given for this semantic change related to the general passivity inferred by the word *patient*. The hope was to avoid (through the use of a different label) the implication that change would come through the efforts of a skilled professional staff rather than by the individual's personal involvement. It was an attempt to give the individual a greater sense of dignity. In effect, however, it supported the patient's denial that there was anything wrong with him. He believed that he was only a transient resident doing his time. Changing the designation without clarifying the actual issues is a deceptive waste of energy. Self-respect comes from the successful accomplishment of personally invested work, not a semantic change.

No Loss Allowed

This is a game primarily seen within the patient population. Frequently, the withdrawal of a particular privilege or reward that has seemed inconsequential causes all the patients to band together and protest that they are undergoing a major loss. In our experience, the patients well understood that some particular behavior would mean the loss of the reward or privilege. There was no apparent reaction to the information when presented. It was only at the moment that the loss was imminent that a reaction occurred.

> *Patients' version:* A pet dog cared for by one of the patients began to look sickly and less vigorous following the departure of this patient. Although another patient and his group had accepted the responsibility of the dog's care, they apparently were not following through on their agreement. The staff brought this up on several occasions, but there was no response. When the staff felt that the dog's health was being jeopardized and that no one was caring for him, they decided that the animal must finally be removed from the unit.
>
> In spite of the fact that many of the group had said they didn't like the dog and, in fact, mistreated him, they all demonstrated and signed a petition strongly protesting the loss.
>
> The reason seemed related to the men's personal sense of emptiness. The object in jeopardy is of little consequence; it is the issue of one's right to decide and possess. When the men share this sense of deprivation, any loss becomes extremely important. They do not seem to respond to the verbal warning of future loss because they have little investment in words as actually conveying planned actions and little concern for the future. But when a loss is imminent, they respond!

Do as I Say, Not as I Do

This game is played by staff or patient. It exhibits the belief that one is exempt from the rules one espouses. One is "specially" privileged. It may be seen in such a small thing as being late to meetings one has urged others to attend promptly.

> *Staff's version:* At one point the patients were asked not to alter or destroy hospital property. They were also

requested not to make window curtains out of sheets. It was learned that the staff members requesting that these sheets not be used had previously acquired them for the patients with this exact purpose in mind.

Patients' version: A resident leader who had been found having intercourse with a woman in the basement had repeatedly made announcements at unit meetings asking the men not to break the rules regarding social restrictions for women.

As long as a person feels entitled to insist on rules but holds that they do not apply to him personally, no progress can be made. Nobody can function in a system with double standards.

Going Through the Motions

Sometimes an alteration in behavior is achieved after a struggle. Following a brief period of apparent success, the spirit goes out of it although the alteration continues to be evident.

This occurs when change is externally motivated or coerced without the genuine involvement of those participating. Overtly, the message is one of compliance, "We will do what you ask." Covertly, the message is another triumph of negativsim, "You can force us to do what you ask, but you cannot force us to think, believe, or feel differently. You cannot force us to be personally invested!"

Because of this game, it is necessary to work out disagreements prior to the inception of any program and to work them out with all concerned. *Individual changes and programs can be successful when all of those involved have participated in the planning, have worked out their differences, and support the proposed alteration.*

> *Staff's version:* A special treatment unit was established for patients who normally would have been dropped from the program to return to prison. Staff members carried out their agreed-upon tasks; however, few expended the extra energy and interest necessary to make this project succeed. Later, one of the staff members explained her lack of interest: "Why should I bother? You and

L. (the unit chief) just rammed it down our throats—so you
take care of it. It's your baby!"

There had been many discussions prior to the establishment of the special unit. Everyone was aware that
the staff harbored a great deal of unspoken resistance. The
unit chief and I became angry at the passive resistance and
decided to go ahead with the plan. Had we taken more
time to resolve the resistance, the project might have succeeded.

Patient–staff's version: The patients, who had previously done almost no work in the unit, were asked to
work 20 hours per week. This demand was based upon the
idea that they needed regular interaction with staff and
peers in a real work situation. The hospital had multiple in-
dustries that provided a work setting not unlike those to be
found outside of the hospital.

Initially, there was great patient resistance to this idea.
Following a struggle in which it became clear that the staff
would use its authority to force the change, there was a
brief swelling of excitement as the men began working
regularly at jobs. When the novelty wore off, a routine developed. Basically, the men were not interested in the
work. They merely went through the motions. They had no
personal goal other than to fulfill the requirement to stay in
the program. They viewed the new therapeutic goal of interaction and work experience as a mere rationalization for
the staff to impose its will. Thus, they could maintain their
view of being "victims" of others' will, while the staff could
feel frustrated and maintain their view of seeing addicts as
unchangeable.

In addition to force and compliance, there are other
factors complicating this kind of interaction. Frequently,
there is the hope that some new endeavor will produce a
quick or dramatic change, obviating the need for long and
difficult work and producing a transient sense of novelty
and excitement. Unfortunately, there are no shortcuts.

False Optimism

Staff members play this game with patients who are polite
and energetic and who seemingly share the same values as the

staff. Such a patient usually presents himself in this agreeable way at the time of first contact or shortly thereafter. The staff members note this and talk about him as a good candidate for re-habilitation. He seems to share their values! Frequently, such a person becomes a leader and urges other patients in a positive direction. This model patient is usually not trying to be decep-tive. He believes that his problems are solved or nonexistent and that he would do better to help others. Staff members over-look his past history and fail to notice that being a leader has frequently allowed him to avoid self-scrutiny. This frequently happens in community and self-help programs that use ex-addicts and ex-convicts.

We dealt with a number of men who functioned this way in Lexington. Each time, we learned that they had always been pleasing to authority. At the same time, they retained the capac-ity for self-destruction. Thus, their model behavior did not rep-resent a change, merely a temporary emphasis on previously available skills. One man who behaved this way gave an earlier history of stealing mail on the same day that he received a 4-H award of merit. He was arrested by the FBI 16 hours after receiving this honor. He did not see the incongruity of his be-havior.

Within the confines of the hospital, these patients usually became involved in episodes in which the model aspects of their behavior gave way to a brief revelation of their self-destructive potential. Repeatedly, staff members failed to deal with these episodes. The reason lay in their desire to maintain the image of someone they could feel hopeful about with regard to drug ab-stinence. They were afraid to deal with the briefly demonstrated pathology for fear of seeing the man as more troubled than he seemed. The optimism served a need within the staff to have ev-idence that gratifying change was possible.

When the staff was able to overcome the pattern of avoid-ance and to confront such individuals, more realistic change be-came apparent. Similarly, the patients would use the same op-timism in viewing themselves. When faced with evidence of character deficiency that had remained unchanged, they would point to unrelated or minor gains in other areas. Overtly, they were saying, "Don't you see that this means that I'm all better and don't have to worry?" Less obvious was the plea that the deficiency was too painful to look at: "Please let me fool myself so I can remain temporarily comfortable."

Summary

The games described above all appear to be variations of the same game, mutual self-deception to avoid discomfort. They are listed separately to provide a focus on the various guises in which they appear.

Although games can be viewed as a system for manipulation and one-upmanship, the goal of help must not be one-upmanship on the part of the helper. The patient is already massively depressed and failing. He does not need to experience a struggle in which the person allegedly helping him is devaluing him.

The therapist's goal should be to ally himself with those elements of the patient's personality that resist the self-destructive urges, however weakly. His first step is to limit the patient's ability to project motivation and responsibility to forces outside himself. As he loses his ability to blame others, he becomes angry, irritable, and finally depressed. The depression is desirable from the therapist's point of view, because it represents the patient's beginning awareness that it is he who is responsible for his current, past, and future status. As he learns that he has always been responsible and can understand himself, the therapist helps him to develop the tools of good judgment and decision making. Depression that occurs in a supportive treatment setting can be usefully understood and resolved. Masked depressions that go unrecognized (addiction, criminality) act like a cancer, slowly destroying the individual.

The therapist and the patient can begin to explore the roots of the patient's sense of futility. Through examination they may learn whether the patient's early premises about himself are now valid. New alternatives are developed and unknown skills found.

Being able to share the painful burden of self-doubt with another human being who does not gloss over them establishes the basis for a new expectation—that perhaps the patient is not so worthless: "If he (the therapist) can talk of this with me and not avoid it, maybe he feels I am not hopeless." When a painful issue is avoided, it confirms to the individual involved that the issue is useless to discuss. It is hopeless. *Open and thoughtful discussion of the most painful issues conveys a realistic sense of hope!!*

CHAPTER 6

Violence*

Frequently ignored in drug programs and prison reform groups is the addict's or prisoner's lack of apparent concern toward his violent or impulsive behavior. Among treatment personnel, there seem to be two extreme views. One, currently not in vogue, is that these individuals are unchangeable, dangerous persons who should be locked away from society forever. The other view disregards the real potential for violence and gives these individuals complete, uncritical, and unquestioning acceptance, without which they allegedly cannot be changed.

In order for any program to be successful, its staff must accept the fact that impulsive, destructive, and violent behavior must not be ignored.

> *Example 1:* Following a group meeting in the clinical research center at Lexington in which a visitor and I had participated, the visitor remarked that the men must genuinely like me in order to be so open with me and each other. (At this time, the group was dealing with racial issues and fears of homosexual assault. These topics are generally too explosive to be explored in prisonlike settings, but there was sufficient group structure to support exploration of

---

* Special thanks to Dr. E. Khantzian for discussions which helped in the writing of this chapter.

these issues.) In response to the visitor's comment, I invited him to return to the group the following day. During the course of the meeting, I asked one of the group members how he would respond if he and I met outside of the center and if I possessed something that he wanted. The man responded with a surprised look, "Oh, you know that one, Doc. I'd take it. If need be, I'd take you out (kill you), but you know, it's nothing personal, I kind of like you!" For this man, business was business. In his experience, murder, assault, and robbery were activities not dependent upon one's feeling for the victim. Because this and other differences in behavioral standards were openly acknowledged, the group could explore the motivations of behavior without the need for evasion and deception.

It was my belief that if the motivation was clear, the destructive option frequently made no sense. Some of the men could give up destructive behavior, not because of changed moral convictions but because they saw their current mode of behavior as personally unprofitable. They found real alternatives that satisfied their needs without the need for violence.

When this genuine inclination to violence is openly clarified, staff must explore the consequences of these forms of behavior within the treatment program and treatment relationship. Frequently, a clear statement of these consequences is sufficient to avert the destructive behavior. In general, it is best to talk about sanctions that depend upon the system in which the individual is working. By and large, threats of legal sanctions and imprisonment are meaningless to these men. Their experience with the legal system has demonstrated a basic hypocrisy: An individual commits an act that he knows to be illegal. If apprehended, he may be able to make a deal with law enforcement officers whereby giving information or other services, he can avoid or minimize the consequences of his actions. Should he be charged and brought before a judge, a lawyer is hired or appointed to aid him in obtaining the least possible legal sanctions for his actions. Frequently, none of the individuals involved—arresting officer, judge, prosecutor, or lawyer—has devoted time to assessing the rehabilitative needs of the particular individual. They are all aware of the backlog of similar cases and lack of effective rehabilitative facilities. Thus, a routine develops that resembles an assembly line, in which the person who has committed the crime is numbered, tagged, and shuttled off. No one in the system believes that any of the available and overcrowded facilities will in any way help the criminal to reenter society in a useful manner. From start to finish, the criminal is enmeshed in a system that verbally espouses help and corrective change, yet is in no way able to provide it. It is a colossal con. He learns that his real crime is getting caught and putting himself at the mercy of a hypocritical system.

Where a legal sanction represents a *realistic* threat, other results can occur.

> *Example 2:* One evening, a doctor was called to see a patient on a psychiatric ward at a private hospital. The patient had been sent by the courts for an evaluation prior to standing trial. That evening he had been threatening patients and staff with physical harm if they would not give in to his demands. There was nothing psychotic in his thinking or behavior. After several minutes of listening to his demands and threats, the physician told him (1) that he was not crazy and had complete responsibility for his behavior; (2) that any attempt to act out his threats would result in additional charges of assault and battery; and (3) that the physician would lodge these charges and had no objection to completing his evaluation of this man within the confines of a jail.
>
> Startled, the patient said, "But Doctor, you are supposed to understand these things, my problems." The physician then told him that an attempt to understand the origin of his behavior did not give him a license to act without responsibility for his actions. A phone call from the hospital later that evening revealed that the young man had stopped his threatening actions and had gone around apologizing to those whom he had previously been terrorizing. He did this not out of any change of heart but for fear of returning to the jail from which he had been sent.

The misconception that individuals in the helping professions are expected to listen, to understand, and to accept abuse
without question is one that has been fostered by both professionals and the popular media. Dynamic psychiatry, with its
wide latitude in the treatment of the neurotic and the psychotic,
was never conceived of as directly applicable to the needs of
people with impulse and character problems.

It is true that the same dynamic understanding is a necessary prerequisite for planning adequate treatment. It does not
mean that the helper should make himself the object of disrespect and abuse. A helper's lack of self-respect in any form of
treatment is most injurious to the patient. Persons with character problems need to see the helper as a model. If he is arbitrary
and capricious, or self-effacing and easily manipulated, the patient will not respect him and will not be able to use him adequately as a model. (Remember the need for the missing
parents.)

> *Example 3:* Earlier, I described an outpatient clinic for
> addicts who were primarily veterans. In addition to metha-
> done treatment, it had a wide-ranging program of individ-
> ual and group therapy, job counseling, and vocational train-
> ing. Part of the requirement for admission was evidence
> that the individual had a serious commitment to changing
> his pattern of living.
>
> Upon entering the building one day, I noted a number
> of patients lounging on the stairs, including the man whom
> I was supposed to see in a consultation. As the conference
> began, I asked, "Has anybody asked this man how lounging
> in the stairwell contributes to his helping himself?" Star-
> tled, his counselor responded, "Oh, I couldn't do that, he'd
> punch me. . . . you don't know, they all carry guns and
> knives."
>
> Almost immediately, other staff members spoke up
> and described threats and situations wherein the men had
> implied that they would harm the staff or the center.
> Frequently, this had been couched in a statement to the in-
> dividual counselor: "I'm only telling you this because I like
> you and want you to get out of here in time." The spontane-

ity of these responses and the barely concealed anxiety were a surprise. The provocative bravado of the men lounging on the stairs began to make sense. The staff and the patients were involved in a silent struggle for control, and the staff was losing!

The staff were then asked to describe their conception of treatment. The counselor who had spoken first stated, "We were taught that these men have been deprived of love and understanding. We are supposed to try and give that, by understanding their needs." This seemed to be a superficial rationalization, an attempt to conceal the fear of confronting unacceptable behavior. *No one can be taught to respect or love himself by being invited to abuse and denigrate his victim–helper.* These patients despise their victim–helpers for their weakness. They are frightened by their victims' helplessness because they fear that this could happen to them. For them, there can be only the superior con man and the despised sucker. If they are to obtain help in any way, they must learn that there are real, viable alternatives to being the abuser and being the abused. Staff members must demonstrate these alternative modes. There can be no treatment where either therapist or patient has a bona fide fear of real violence in the treatment situation.

Before presenting the case, we discussed the idea that love might mean saying *no* to unreasonable demands and refusing to accept abuse. It was clear that the loving parent has to say no, to set limits, to discipline the growing child. This needs to be done empathically, not punitively.

The conference then began. The man who was going to be discussed had been home from Vietnam for 2 years. He had been in trouble as a juvenile offender prior to entering the service. He lived at home with his mother and came to the clinic several times a week. He had been a machinist in the service, and the staff wanted to know whether to set up a shop in the outpatient clinic in order to give this man a work experience. In his 2 years in the program, he had not worked and frequently used opiates and barbiturates. Staff members liked this man but felt unable to help him. They viewed him as a man stuck in a position dependent upon both the clinic and his mother for his survival. As we explored the idea of the shop, the man's daily routine became clear. He spent part of his time in the clinic going from counselor to counselor in unscheduled appointments, having "heart-to-heart" talks. Part of the time he spent out in the streets. It was then mentioned that he was reputed to be one of the largest drug dealers in the area. He had been sought for many months by various dissatisfied customers and was constantly under threat of violence and death.

This "poor, dependent man" who was so incapable of caring for himself was in fact an energetic and resourceful person who daily negotiated a dangerous life dealing with customers and middlemen and avoiding police and a number of enemies. This view of his behavior as energetic and skilled had been ignored. In fact, the man had considerable adaptive strengths.

Another incident then came to light. Several weeks prior to the conference the patient had beaten up his mother. Like the staff at the clinic, she too had refused to deal with his behavior and had allowed him to continue living at home with no expectations from him. This continued acceptance of his behavior without question or expectation of change was very destructive. At one level, it confirmed his view that suckers are born to be taken advantage of. After all, wasn't his mother a sucker? At another level, by accepting him the way he was, his mother raised several questions in his mind: "Is this all I am? Is that all I can be? Do I really need to be coddled this way? Can't anyone expect more of me? Am I so bad or so different from other people that no one can deal with me directly, no matter how provocative I am?"

In reviewing the incident with his mother, the staff had accepted the patient's statement that he couldn't remember any of the assault on his mother because he had experienced a "blackout." Repeated questioning in the conference revealed that he did remember purposely assaulting his mother. A blackout had occurred after the assault had begun and seemed to be an unconsciously motivated protection by which the patient ultimately prevented himself from murdering his mother. He fainted and could not complete the assault. He was both frightened and ashamed of his attack. His hostile, but dependent and loving, relationship was threatened by the emergence of feelings of rage toward his mother.

These were feelings that he neither understood nor adequately contained. The inability of the staff to deal with behavior that was clearly visible gave him no confidence that he could reveal the even more troubling rage that he had felt during the assault. He had no experience to teach him that he and other people could tolerate knowing his inner emotional experience and deal with it.

As this material emerged in the conference, the patient became furious and menacing toward me. He said that he would like to drop me out of the window and watch me land on the pavement below, smashed and bleeding.

This statement drew several questions in response. Did he really believe I would then come to feel some of the internal pain that he was experiencing? What did he imagine I would look like as I lay bleeding and battered on the pavement? The questions brought forth tearful memories of the maimed and discarded bodies of friends that the patient had seen in Vietnam. By the pursuing of imagery that was frightening to the patient and the interviewer, another painful area emerged for investigation and resolution. He was no longer alone with painful memories and feelings.

At the end of the conference, I made several recommendations. A two-part program was designed, the first part defining the expectation that the patient would work and attend the program in a regular way. This would be coupled with an assessment of his day-to-day behavior and its implications. Much of the assessment would be conducted in group meetings. Words and promises would not be allowed to outweigh behavior. For the second part, painful experiences would be explored to determine the origins of his fears and impulses; this could be done simultaneously in individual and group sessions. Thus, a balanced program was designed, one part dealing with current behavioral needs and the other with the origins of the disruptive behavior. Both programs needed to be carried out simultaneously.

For the clinic, I recommended that the staff decide

reasonable expectations and clear definitions of their limits within the program. Once they had done this, a similar clarification had to be made for the patients.

The staff met and worked out what they believed to be reasonable expectations of behavior, respect, and evidence of investment in the program. These included no lounging about the center, involvement in jobs or scholastic programs, and the closing of the center game rooms. Violence and the threat of violence were not to be tolerated in the program. This prohibition and the consequences were clearly defined. Regular methadone hours were established. There was no place for other drugs while a patient was in the treatment program, and the consequences of breaking this rule were defined. After this plan had been in effect for the clinic at large for 2 weeks, the same counselor who initially feared being punched stated, "Things are really going well. It's much more relaxed around here. The men seem more comfortable. It's as if they are less upset too." Indeed, this was true. The patients' anxiety about being out of control had been increased by the staff's inability to deal with behavior that the patients themselves knew was unreasonable. This situation is familiar to people who have raised children. When a child's behavior seems to be out of control, an adult is needed to step in and stop it. The child calms down and seems to be relieved. *If he is left unattended, there is a steady escalation of his lack of control; the individual needs the reassurance that he will not be allowed to injure himself or others by an explosion of uncontrolled emotion.*

Destructiveness Outside of Treatment

Destructive behavior is frequently overlooked on the grounds that it occurs outside the program. By ignoring events outside the treatment setting, staff members say that they do not wish to interfere with the right of the patient to a private life. While a person's need for privacy is clear, this is no bar to a staff member's evaluating the individual's life away from the treatment setting in order to ascertain whether he is genuinely extending the treatment work into his daily life.

Example. While consulting in a private drug-treatment program, a colleague was asked how he would deal with the following situation: A program member had been involved in a fight in which two men had been stabbed. When some of the staff members discussed it with the individual informally, he told them that he really had been defending another friend. The staff was divided on whether this was an issue for their concern. Some felt that this incident had to be evaluated, while others believed that since it had occurred outside the center it was a private affair.

As the details emerged, it turned out that the program member and his friend had been attacked by two individuals who were known troublemakers. The four had been sitting together drinking for several hours when the fight occurred. One group of staff members blamed everything on the two troublemakers and wanted to end the discussion. Other staff members and the consultant disagreed. Why had the man in the program been drinking? "Oh, everyone has a drink once in a while" was the reply. If the group member involved had been as upright as some of the staff seemed to believe, then what kind of judgment was he showing by spending several hours with people known for their propensity for violence and illegal behavior?

There followed some comments that it would be unreasonable to expect a person to change his whole way of life and give up his friends. Yet was it? To associate with these people left the individual open to involvement with many forms of self-destructive behavior. Altering criminal behavior and drug taking is a decision of such major proportions that it does involve making drastic changes in one's way of life. Some of the staff felt that this line of reasoning would mean that they would have to examine all incidents of disruptive behavior. This would be too great a burden. Others felt that they were required to scrutinize all issues and events in order to understand the motivation and judgment behind behavior. As is often the case, there was no unanimous resolution to these conflicting views. The consultant and I believed that all behavior is subject to scrutiny and understanding. Consistency demands it.

The Inherent Nature of Violence

The fact that violence is inherent in the character structure of many (not all) persons addicted to drugs was demonstrated in many ways by the men at Lexington. When a group of 60 men were studied intensively during their stay at Lexington, 15 of them spontaneously stated that they had chosen opiates as an alternative to alcohol. They had done so because their alcohol abuse had led to violent outbursts directed against the women (mothers, wives, and girlfriends) with whom they were living and upon whom they were dependent. One man had stopped himself while strangling his mother; another had stopped himself after cutting his mother's throat. When these data were released to the men, many more came forward, stating that they too had given up alcohol and had chosen opiates because of the connection between their own violent behavior and alcohol. (These additional men were not included in the data because what they said depended too easily on what they had been told.)

Another man told of his association of violence with the need for opiates by telling how anxious, tense, and nervous he felt after shooting two men: "I needed the stuff to calm me down, get in control. I couldn't go around shaking like that."

At one time, close to 20% of the 65 men on a treatment unit at Lexington had clearly implied that they had been involved in murders. Because they were not legally protected, they did not describe the details or directly state that they had committed the murders. However, several individuals who had been acquitted of murders did discuss how they, in fact, had committed these crimes.

So, how does one deal with the pressure of impulses so dangerous and frightening? Here are people who act out impulses that the rest of us have spent years learning to repress. By altering or sublimating this kind of murderous rage, we are able to function in our society. We develop close relationships that arouse intense feelings (both loving and destructive) without fear that they will be acted upon. What happens, then, when we are confronted with people who act on feelings that we contain. I find these experiences personally upsetting and frightening. No amount of repetition relieves this. Whenever I have spent time with individuals who give me the feeling of their capacity for violence and their barely controlled impulses, I go through several painful and frightening internal responses.

For instance, when sitting with some brutal and intelligent murderers, I have wished that they were locked up in stone-walled dungeons or executed. Then, I would be safe from them. At other times, I have found myself briefly charmed by their intelligence or conversation. In that fantasy, I become a special friend or ally. After all, he wouldn't hurt a friend? Nonsense! Such fleeting fantasies and physical sensations of tightness and coldness in the abdomen signal to me that I am deeply frightened. Here sitting with me is someone whom I would wish to appear as a monster. Then the difference between him and me would become all the more apparent. There should be something startling and different to set him apart from me! He has really done the things that I can only barely perceive in fantasy. All of my training and upbringing has led me to abhor real violence and murder. Angry feelings, rage-filled fantasies, yes, but assault and murder, NO! And yet he sits there talking calmly, comfortably. He has murdered and I am uncomfortable, not he! Having explored more deeply at other times what this confrontation touches within me (my own fears of rage and destruction) and having clarified my own responses, I usually proceed to explore the destructive events in the patient's life without the burden of my unreasonable fears.

Once I have accepted into my consciousness that these events have occurred, that this man's frame of reference is different from mine with regard to these acts, we can begin together to understand their origin. If I should try to deny to myself my initial fear of my potential for violence—the potential we all have—I would be unable to consider what issues entered into these acts. I would need to exclude them from my awareness. As will be shown in the story of V. (p. 165), close examination of the origin of behavior can lead to understanding and perhaps change. It cannot be done if the therapist needs to deny his own shock, fear, and revulsion.

Through repeated experiences with such people, it has become apparent to me that one cannot back away from the problems of such individuals without paying a significant price. There are some individuals for whom our resources at this time are insufficient to meet their needs. Permanent incarceration and study may be the only possible mode of coping with them. However, the number of people actually needing such confinement is probably less than those currently incarcerated. Permanent incarceration or execution will eliminate a few potential murderers, but it will not put aside our own fear of the violent potential in ourselves. Similarly, to allow ourselves to be charmed into avoiding direct confrontation of these issues will cause us to pay a personal price of humiliation and danger. One cannot escape the knowledge of what one has avoided, no matter what the rationalization. After going through this kind of thought and evaluation, one proceeds to evaluate the facts of the individual's behavior, with the hope of clarifying with him his motivations.

This personal internal process of denial or identification with an aggressor may be observed in the staff members of all the treatment settings mentioned previously. While most addicts are not murderers, many are consistently violent people. Others use drugs to help in their struggle to control their own violent impulses and feelings. Thus, they may readily communicate a sense of imminent explosiveness to the drug counselor or the therapy group. At such times, the defenses noted above may come into play, as staff members and other patients become apprehensive and seek to allay their anxiety through one of the defenses of avoidance. If this apprehension and its source in the patient's behavior are brought out in the open, anxiety is diminished and change may be effected. If they are avoided, there is no possible change and an escalation occurs that forces someone to set a limit.

Example: A drug counselor gave the following example of a problem patient in his group. The patient had been increasingly provocative and loud in the group, interrupting and shouting at other group members. The counselor at first ignored the patient but on successive occasions was forced to respond. He tried to understand the patient "empathically." The patient described an increasing number of fights and disputes outside the group. Over several weeks, neither the group nor the leader could deal with these events. On one occasion, the patient jumped up, obviously very excited. When the leader asked in his most understanding voice why the man had been so upset, the patient punched him and left the group. He was then excluded and not allowed to return.

A review of the group sessions revealed the following background. The group had been growing cohesive and had developed an ability to look at the depressive issues of loneliness and desperation that this man also experienced. The patient in question had felt increasingly isolated. His outbursts had temporarily stopped the process of group cohesion. The group and the leader had allowed this to occur by not directly acknowledging and confronting his desperation and anxiety. Perhaps, they covertly supported his behavior in order to prevent further anxiety-laden exploration of the group's depressive issues. They were aware of increasing discomfort and the wish that this man would leave the group. They could not directly express their anger and fear and their wish that he would leave. Instead, the group superficially adopted the leader's mode of "empathic understanding." When the patient in question could no longer tolerate this kind of nonresponse to his demonstrated anxiety, he assaulted the group leader and left. One of his subsequent comments to the leader was "I couldn't tolerate it, your steady syrupy stuff."

The patient was not allowed to return to the group or to stay in the program. If his problem had been dealt with earlier, he might have been able to remain and make use of the group process.

By directly discussing observed behavior, the group and the therapists have an opportunity to demonstrate that they are not overwhelmed by the implied violence. They thus reassure the explosive patient that they can contain and explore the distress that leads him to act in such a defensive and hostile manner. As the next example demonstrates, not all violence is shown in gross behavior. Tone of voice, appearance, eye contact, and manner of interaction can convey a menacing quality. In whatever form it appears, violence and its potential need to be acknowledged.

Example: In group therapy in Lexington, a recently admitted man, Hugo, was intimidating the group. He had been acquitted of one murder (which he had in fact committed), and allegedly he had committed six more, as well as a number of other violent assaults upon people. Reports from local agencies in his home town confirmed his reputation. His style of a fixed stare, an expressionless face, and a steady delivery of short, monotone sentences had a chilling effect. At other times, he spoke with a pseudofriendly, jovial quality that was quite eerie.

Another recent admission, an adolescent, Frank, was describing to the group his frightening experience of being gang-raped in prison. Hugo implied sarcastically that Frank had probably asked for it and enjoyed it. In the group were a number of ex-convicts who had raped young boys in prison. In spite of this, they were able to discuss their experience and Frank's in a useful way that did not contain the same criticism and derision as Hugo had shown. When Hugo maintained his sadistic verbal assault, the group leader asked him what was so upsetting to him that he needed to be so destructive. The group became quiet and a few people moved their chairs back. Although there had been no directed threat, the group leader was also frightened. Hugo glowered, smiled slowly, and then delivered a steady and explosive barrage about "fairy psychiatrists." The leader responded by asking if that was one of the worries he had about himself, being a "fairy." Did he really see himself as being so like Frank? At this, Hugo left the group. Later, he asked the group leader for an individual appointment.

At the appointment, he began by apologizing for his

outburst. He began complimenting the leader for his determination and insight. This was flattering groundwork for some conning maneuver, but he was also probing to see if he could have a safer discussion. When the con and flattery were acknowledged, he was asked what he really wanted. He hesitated, then said, "Doc, is it true that the guy who gives it out winds up getting?" This meant, "Is it true that the homosexual assaulter winds up seeking homosexual abuse?" He went on to describe tough men whom he had respected who wound up being slavishly used by weak, effeminate boys. Following this, he described an incident in which a gang of prisoners had cornered him and tried to rape him when he was first imprisoned. Some friends rescued him. Following that, he always acted in a belligerent, sadistic manner while in prison. He participated in several homosexual rapes to demonstrate to others that he was "on top."

Hugo knew that the gist of the meeting would be made known to the group, yet he continued. Was homosexuality hereditary? Questioning revealed that a family member was homosexual. Finally, he described situations in which he had admired and felt close to several men. In each instance, he had ended the relationship by seriously injuring the person he was attracted to. When his longing for closeness became too threatening, he resolved his internal conflict by viciously attacking the other person. He saw the fights as being precipitated by the other person's attempt to make him unmanly: "If I let that guy go, I wouldn't be a man."

He then asked that the conversation be only partially revealed to the group (the purpose of the original flattery). The request was denied. When the discussion was returned to the group, a verbal struggle recurred but the material was brought out. Because the group leader was not intimidated or cajoled into ignoring the issues, the rest of the group addressed Hugo. One of them said, "Man, looking at Frank was like looking in the mirror for you. No wonder you were such a gorilla."

It is noteworthy that Hugo's behavior for the rest of his stay in the hospital showed that he had learned about some of the issues that precipitated his angry outbursts and was bet-

ter able to manage them. He gave up his menacing appearance and style. This would not have happened if the group
had ignored his early behavior. Just prior to discharge he
resumed his previous mode of behavior, as a preparation to
returning to the streets.

As indicated by these two cases, the success of treatment
programs depends upon the staff's capacity to deal with threats
to their own emotional makeup. Many drug programs are staffed
by young, energetic people who have a personal commitment to
"rescuing" the addict. For some, this urge to rescue is related to
a view of the addict as a victim of the society that the helper
wants to change. This sense of purpose with its attendant excitement is a valuable attribute. Yet, it is also a potential hazard.
The addict may perceive that the commitment shown by his
counselor comes from the counselor's personal need and may
resent the "ego trip" of the helper who seems to be overly understanding or excessively interested in some aspect of the addiction experience. He realizes that the counselor is seeing him
as a symbol of his own crusade, not as a real person.

Many counselors come from middle-class environments and
are intrigued by the association with people whose life experience is so violent and unpredictable. A counselor who worked in
one such program reported, "I feel so excited in the program. At
any moment something can happen. There is always danger. It's
nothing like college or home." Fantasies that emerged in the
therapy of this person revealed that the behavior of his patients
in the drug program coincided with the patient–counselor's unconscious desire for violence. The danger to the treatment program arose from the helper's unconscious wish to have the addict continue his destructive behavior as a means of vicariously
satisfying the counselor's needs.

Similarly, there have been many news media stories about
public figures who become transiently enamored with radical or
criminal groups. There are also reports of students from middle-
class and upper-class backgrounds who join with criminal groups
in suicidal coalitions. They are "radicals" who identify genuine

social issues but use them to deal with personal conflicts within themselves. They become easy prey for sociopathic persons who are adept at the rhetoric of social issues but have no illusions of personal commitment to any social beliefs. The alliance is one between the idealist who needs the beliefs to justify his actions and avoid the knowledge of his inner turmoil and the pragmatic criminal who is merely using the current social issues as a conning device for those gullible enough to accept it. The extreme example is that of Charles Manson and his followers.

This internal need and motivation on the part of the helper become crucial in self-help programs that employ or are led by ex-addicts and ex-convicts. There have been a number of instances in which ex-addicts have become leaders and directors of large drug-treatment programs. In each situation, these men were intelligent and articulate people who worked diligently to create viable treatment programs. They developed goals, programs, and philosophies that were based upon the highest ideals and gained wide support in their communities and even nationally. The leaders were widely sought after as speakers to civic and community groups. Each man was a convincing example of addict rehabilitation. In many instances, the close supervision initially provided by a nonaddict director had all but disappeared. No attention was paid to the unresolved destructive elements in the individual's character. He was left to his own devices. (The directors of drug programs frequently become preoccupied with the public relations aspect of their programs and leave the day-to-day work to others. For some program directors, the temptation to gain prestige and power has superseded any earlier interest in drug treatment.)

Many of these leaders subsequently returned to drug abuse, violence, and jail. In one instance, the leader surrounded himself with a group of youths, addicts and nonaddicts alike, who were bound to him by forced experiences of sodomy and torture. In spite of these perverted experiences, some of these young people picketed at his trial, protesting that he was being unfairly maligned by a government plot. At the time of indictment, this self-help unit and the indicted (later convicted) leader were the subject of a laudatory article in a nationally distributed journal. The wish to ignore the unsolved turmoil in these individuals is deleterious to their growth.

In summary, close attention must be paid to the personal motivation of the staff. The helper motivated by high purpose that serves personal needs may overlook the potential for violence and deception in the people with whom he is working. He is likely to say, "What do you expect? That's all he knows how to do." This view of the addict as hopelessly unable to change and irresponsible can be a device to continue the helper's vicarious experience of violence and excitement.

Neither the addict client nor his helper may be aware that changes in behavior and attitude become fixed only when there is a basic change in character. *Changes in character require constant, painful attention over a long time.* There is an urgency in most drug-treatment settings to demonstrate rapid, effective changes. This is closely related to the competitive drive to obtain the limited Federal funding. This need for quick results is at variance with the concept that genuine character change requires continuous work over a prolonged period of time. Without a resolution of this conflict, short-term, less intense programs may predominate and convey the inaccurate conclusion that long-term, effective character change cannot occur: "Once a junky (criminal, etc.), always a junky." The addict leaders previously mentioned were done a disservice when their needs for close evaluation and supervision were ignored. Although these men spoke of lofty ideals, none had ever gone through the intensive treatment experiences that they asked of others. Their previously available intelligence and skills were utilized to deny their personal treatment needs. Their program directors were pleased with the prospect of having such individuals, who could be publicly marketed as examples of highly motivated ex-addicts. They overlooked the fact that none had shown evidence of working through the slow process of character change. They collaborated with their program directors in a mutually destructive exploitation: "I'll make your program look good if you'll leave me alone." The addict or convict who is given a responsibility without adequate supervision will act in his usual way. The same holds true for the staff.

A summary of the points made in this chapter may be useful.

1. Fear of violence is an experience common to *all* drug programs.

2. When this fear is inadequately dealt with, the program falters.

3. There is a primary failure of identification of this fear, which involves rationalization, denial, suppression, and identification with the aggressor.

4. When this occurs, the patient can intimidate and blackmail his would-be helpers.

5. The patient becomes more anxious as his helpers and fellow patients retreat before his threats. The impulses that he believes to be uncontrollable become the governing factor. His experience with those about him supports his fear that these impulses are uncontrollable. He then panics and precipitates a crisis that must be dealt with.

6. Most addicts have character defects having to do with the integration of violence and aggression into their personality in an adaptive manner. Treatment programs must recognize this and reflect it back to the addict. The patient must learn to recognize his personal problem with violent impulses and see the program as steadily attuned to it and working with it.

7. Even the most experienced and insightful ex-addict needs continued attention to these issues over time. Failure to give him this attention is tantamount to abandoning him to an isolated position where he finds it necessary to hide the very problems that he is helping others to deal with. This abandonment and isolation contribute to the failure of many ex-addicts who had genuinely been motivated to alter their lives.

8. Drug-addict and convict rehabilitation programs attract staff members who are struggling with intense personal needs. If these needs go unaddressed, the programs fail in their stated aims. Staff members must be able to deal with their own conflicts before they can effectively assist their clients. Frequently,

this requires identifying personal needs, altering ideals, and recognizing cultural and experiential differences. Staff and patients must give up fantasies of quick alteration and of rescuing clients as a means of solving their own personal problems.

9. It is necessary to recognize that genuine change requires long-term treatment that constantly deals with behavior, motivation, and attitude. Dramatic, short-term gains are frequently short in duration.

CHAPTER 7

A Graphic Approach
to Understanding
Intrapersonal Processes

Many persons fail to understand the role of their emotions and defenses in the origin of their own behavior. Frequently, the person with a destructive character disorder is unaware of the causes of his actions. He reacts without thought. Because of this lack of personal awareness, he can remain free of the anxiety, depression, and panic that are related to his internal doubts and conflicts. He tends to explain his behavior solely in terms of superficial and external circumstances. Such explanations absolve him of any personal responsibility for failure.

When this person confronts a professional helper whose investment lies in understanding behavior in terms of internal drives and other determinants rather than external causes, his defenses are automatically galvanized to resist this threatening perspective.

There are other factors that interfere with the formation of a working relationship between the patient and the counselor. The patient views the counselor's education and professional skills with distrust. The patient uses action to deal with prob-

155

lems; the counselor uses observation, reconstruction, and understanding. The patient frequently views the counselor as a dangerous con man. Many patients have avoided eye contact with me and later have explained to me that they felt that my training and background would allow me to read their minds. Once I knew their most private thoughts they feared that I would use them to humiliate the individual. Such magical beliefs and fantasies are compatible with the developmental theory in Chapter 4.

In numerous situations, I have seen the patient fail to relate a present happening to previous experiences. When the patient was able to see clearly that he was repeating a previous experience, the effect upon him was dramatic. Where I felt compelled to resort to complicated or vague and theoretical explanations, the concept was poorly understood and the result was increased distrust. From this it became evident that a concept is meaningful to both the person speaking and the listener only when it can be clearly and simply stated. As a result, I developed the graphic approach to helping the patient to obtain some objective distance in viewing himself and his interactions with the environment. Behavior, feelings, traits, and interactions become clear through the use of the schematic approach mentioned in Chapter 4 and further developed here.

As noted earlier, patients distrust everyone, including their comrades. They view the world as an unsafe environment in which others are always trying to take them off guard and use them. Alleged helpers with different educational, racial, religious, and cultural backgrounds are more dangerous because they operate in a different frame of reference than one's comrades. As one man described, "I always feel more comfortable in prison. I know who and what I am. I don't have to fool anyone. I'm just a thief and con man and that's all anyone expects." His anxiety is diminished because he has a defined role that he is familiar with.

In treatment settings, the anxiety increases because there is an expectation on the part of the would-be counselor that the individual can be more than he has allowed himself to be. The patient is busy trying to find a way to define and fit in most comfortably to the helper's expectations without changing or expending energy. He is anxious until he learns the helper's "game" and has found a "safe" response. I found that introducing the graphic system helped to reduce the patient's initial discomfort. It helped the patient understand the concept of personal identity and provided the patient and the therapist with a mutual external focus in the form of a shared activity. This activity was filling in the schematic picture.

Patient, therapist, and therapy group participated in observing behavior, guessing at its meaning, and writing in the information. Eye-to-eye contact was intermittent as the attention was focused on the blackboard or paper. Disagreements included all group participants and did not focus only on the person or people under discussion. Thus, the individual felt less as if he was isolated while under scrutiny. Arguments between individuals centered on what words were to be written in the scheme or where an idea was to be included. This seemed to diminish the sense of personal threat. One could say that the externalization (writing on the blackboard) made use of the addict's common defense of displacement and projection outside of himself. This reduced the defensive quality of the interchange and increased the patient's interest in the process.

This gimmicklike introduction of the blackboard and schema reduced tension and increased interest because of its novelty. The initial seduction via use of novelty seemed to enhance the result to the patient—a concise, comprehensive view of himself, his behavior, its motivation, and its origin. Additionally, it added a view of himself with a time perspective—a continuum of past and present.

In short, drawing a picture made it possible for the patient to take something concrete from therapy. The men spontaneously copied down the completed drawing and began reworking it. It became a useful device to review a therapy session. *Frequently, they could not rely on their own memories because their defenses automatically concealed from them the painful issues that the group had elicited.* They discussed the idea in the

schema with group members or the therapist after a session as
they reworked the concept it contained. The drawing was initially used in group settings. Later, drawings were found to be
useful with couples and adolescents in family settings. They
seemed to provide a kind of external focus in situations in which
emotions were running too high to allow for direct observation.
The schema was needed less as the individual began to tolerate
more direct personal assessment. The technique was used primarily in the first months of treatment only.

Figures 5 and 6 review the diagrams of Chapter 4. Figure 5
shows the individual as the rectangular figure. To his left is the
space representing his current reality. To the right of the rectangle is the space representing his developmental input.

Within the individual there are two subdivisions. The left

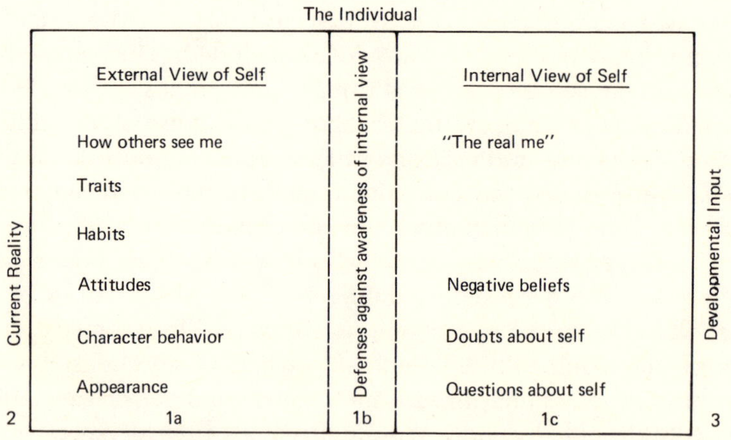

The Individual

	External View of Self	Defenses against awareness of internal view	Internal View of Self	
Current Reality	How others see me		"The real me"	Developmental Input
	Traits			
	Habits			
	Attitudes		Negative beliefs	
	Character behavior		Doubts about self	
	Appearance		Questions about self	
2	1a	1b	1c	3

Part 1a, the left side of the rectangle reflects the appearance the individual hopes
to convey to the world about him.
Part 1b, reflects the defenses against full awareness by the individual of his personal doubts and beliefs about himself.
Part 1c, pictures the individual's internal view of himself. This view is generally
avoided by the individual and hidden from those about him.
Part 2, the space to the left of Figure, represents events and influences in the individual's current reality that impinge upon him.
Part 3, the space to the right of Figure, represents the area of developmental
influences that impinged on him in the past.

Figure 5

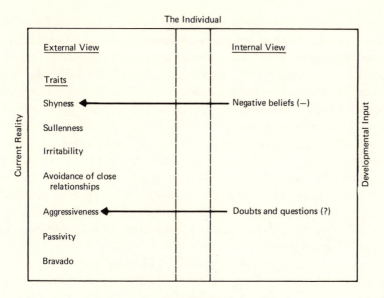

Figure 6

side represents the external self or the self he shows to the
world. This area contains his traits, observable habits, manner-
isms, behavior, etc. The right side of the rectangle contains the
internal self. This part the individual hides from others and
frequently from his own awareness. The two are kept separate
by defenses represented by the broken double line.

When an individual has succeeded in repressing or sup-
pressing a particular self-doubt or negative belief, one usually
finds evidence of its existence in his attitudes, actions, and character traits. This partial expression of the obscured issues is
represented by the arrows in Figure 6. These defenses function
imperfectly, thus the broken lines.

The impulsive individual generally views his behavior as
being motivated by the environment. He views himself as a victim forced to react to protect himself (Figure 7). He acknowledges no internal motivation for his behavior.

The fact is that an individual's response is frequently out of
proportion to the environmental incidents. This disparity be-

tween input and response can become the wedge that helps to draw the individual's attention to factors within himself. Many times an individual would become interested when the disproportionate response was noted and deemed "foolish." To the therapist, it was clear that some internal doubt or conflict had been touched. The anxiety aroused was dealt with by an excessive defensive response, developed to protect the individual from some inner pain. Unable to tolerate self-observation and discomfort, the individual automatically mobilized his defenses to reduce the anxiety, depression, or pain.

The exaggerated quality represents the degree of internal conflict and an attempt to localize outside of the individual (Figure 8). This mechanism involves projection, denial, distortion, and projective identification.

These are relatively primitive defenses that have never been abandoned in favor of more mature ones. Usually, the defenses contain the doubts and negative beliefs. Under increased pressure, the individual may use alcohol, other substances, or distracting behavior to reinforce the defenses. Under excessive pressure or in acute situations, the primitive explosion occurs. Such people are walking bombs.

The large arrow in Figure 8 represents this primitive defense. It is an attempt to externalize the internal doubt that seems to threaten the individual. In that sense, it can be called a

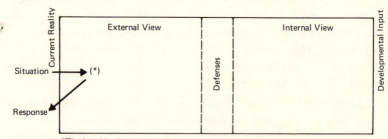

*The inpulsive individual's view of his responses. Note that he denies the existence of his defense, internal motivations, and past. He also sees his response as proportionate.

Figure 7

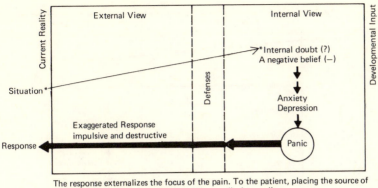

The response externalizes the focus of the pain. To the patient, placing the source of the discomfort outside of his inner-self has a relieving quality.

Figure 8

projective defense. The initial issue is distorted and is perceived as a statement by the external source that the individual is exactly what he has always feared himself to be. More simply, the person reacts as if someone else is stating that all those negative beliefs about himself are true: "You're saying I'm worthless." Instead of going into an examination of the internal doubt, all energy goes into denial, projection, and a retaliatory defense aimed at eliminating the doubt as represented by the outside threat.

If the personal doubts or negative beliefs are known to the patient, we speak of them as conscious. If his defenses make him unaware of the doubts or negative beliefs, we speak of them as unconscious. Someone suffering from unconscious negative beliefs speaks in general terms of poorly defined discomfort, irritability, and vague feelings of unease. Example 1, Figure 9, clarifies the usefulness of the diagram system.

Example 1: Ralph was 38 years old when he was seen at a drug treatment center for multiple drug abusers. He was conditionally admitted to the program as an alternative to returning to jail for parole violations. He had a 25-year history of drug usage and 17 years of incarceration.

At first, he was sullen and hostile, commenting that we

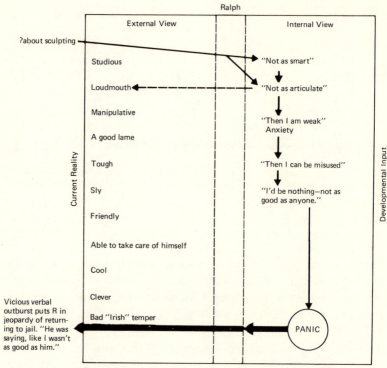

The quote "He was saying, like I wasn't as good as him" represents the projected internal doubt.

Figure 9

would just string him along and then send him to the "joint." Observations of him in the treatment milieux revealed that he could be humorous, engaging, and intelligent. Periodically, this large, red headed, self-caricatured "Irishman" would explode into menacing rages. When questioned about these episodes, he would explain them as mere reactions to external provocations. Was there anything more personal being touched in these incidents?

"No man, what you see is what there is. It's only my Irish temper."

"Perhaps, but this so-called Irish temper could put you back in jail."

As incidents began to occur with greater frequency and

Ralph's behavior jeopardized his stay in the center, we tried to understand the origins of the behavior in his treatment group. Ralph maintained that he was an uncomplicated simple person whose personality could be understood by the characterizations noted in the left side of the rectangle in Figure 5. Examination of one of these outbursts did lead to some clarification of the situation.

Ralph was in the occupational therapy room working on a sculpture. Another patient, Bill, wandered in and casually inquired of Ralph, what he was doing. Ralph did not answer and Bill repeated his question. Ralph turned suddenly on Bill, brandishing a chisel, he cursed and swore. Bill retreated from Ralph's threats indicating that he thought Ralph was crazy. When pushed for an explanation in group, Ralph tried to joke and attribute it to his "Irish temper" saying he meant nothing by it. The group would not accept this explanation and pressed Ralph further. Seeing that neither humor nor apologies would smooth it over, Ralph retreated into a sullen silence. Explosive outbursts, threats, and brandishing weapons would not be tolerated. Any further incidents and Ralph would have to leave the center and go back to court. As this was clarified, Ralph said "Look, he (Bill) was acting superior, like I wasn't as good as him." We tried to diagram Ralph's character and the response.

Ralph and the group easily filled in the area labeled "external view." With minimum discussion and some good-humored banter Ralph agreed with the characterization of himself as: a loudmouth, manipulative, a good, "lame," tough, sly, friendly, able to take care of himself, cool, clever, and having "a bad Irish temper." A seemingly incongruous trait was also noted. He was studious at the center and in prison. Ralph attended classes and took correspondence courses.

Yet, none of these characteristics explained Ralph's disproportionate response to Bill. The group picked up on this and Ralph's studiousness. By way of explanation, Ralph stated that during his first incarceration one of the older more respected prisoners had turned to Ralph and said: "You're an ignorant, stupid, no-account jackass."

"That man could talk circles around me, I felt like a

fool and in the joint guys (speaking to group) you don't want to feel like a fool!"

With this statement Ralph hoped to explain his status and close the issue. He became uncomfortable as we continued to discuss it. He anxiously stated that he felt he "wasn't as smart" and "couldn't speak so good." Because of his visible anxiety we wrote: "not as smart" and "not as articulate" under internal view of Figure 5. The therapist wondered what it was like to feel you were not as smart and could not speak as well as others. Ralph quickly glanced at the therapist and Bill. With a mixture of tension and anger he blurted out: "It means you're *weak*!" Spontaneously, in a pressured manner, he continued:

"To be a good con man, one has to be skillful and intellectually superior. Without that you're weak!"

And, if you were *weak* in the streets?

"Man, you would be misused"

And, if, you were misused?

"I'd be nothing, not as good as anyone!" (looking furious)

We were amazed. Ralph's words had tumbled out amid a rush of powerful feelings. He had stated that his inner fear "being nothing," being *not as good as another* person was what he had heard in Bill's innocuous question. He was reminded of Bill's exact words and his explanation. Quite literally, he had externalized his self-doubt and attributed it to Bill (psychologic defense of projection, and projective identification). He then could vent his rage toward what he perceived as an external threat.

We then focused upon Bill. He was more articulate than Ralph and occasionally did act superior. The occupational therapist and other witnesses to the incident familiar with both Ralph and Bill did not see Bill as acting superior in that incident. The occupational therapist did note that Bill was skilled with his hands and had just completed an intricate hanging mobile. Ralph had been aware of this and talked about being self-conscious about his first attempt at sculpture, which he felt was not going well.

With these issues clarified, Ralph and the group could see that he was reliving earlier humiliations and fears of

being weak and controlled by others. His constant mouth-
ing off was seen as an attempt to force people to acknowledge his presence and authority: "I am somebody" and "I
am not weak."

Subsequently, Ralph was able to deal with his tendency for outbursts. When people saw that he was building
toward an explosion, they were able to interrupt it by asking: "Why do you feel so small in these circumstances?"
Ralph copied down the schema of Figure 5 and returned to
discuss it frequently with his therapist. Although simplified
and failing to explain much in his character, it was a useful
means to approach his behavior. It meant that there was
something to be understood. Events just did not happen.
At a two-year follow-up, Ralph was working and not in jail.
He certainly has not changed and has many character problems, yet he periodically writes to the author to try and further understand his behavior.

Behavioral episodes provided many of the initial situations
that the groups and individuals could explore. Frequently, they
became quite complicated to the outsider, but they were clear
to the participants. Example 2 demonstrates the graphic system
as it begins to include experience, developmental influences,
and cultural factors. Racism and its accompanying devaluation,
combined with poverty, family disorganization, and despair, become developmental influences.

Example 2: Vic was a 28-year-old black high school
dropout. He was born and raised in the poor section of a
moderate-sized northern city. His family was large and
under constant financial stress. He entered a treatment
center after being acquitted of homicide. His mood fluc-
tuated from superficial friendliness to a cool hostility. He
presented himself as an angry black nationalist who was
sensitive to any real or inferred racial slight. He justified all
of his outbursts as resulting from external circumstances.
Several incidents, however, helped uncover his internal
viewpoint.

During a therapy session, the group focused upon a

serious argument that had resulted in a fight. Vic and Paul (another angry black man) were dividing up the cleaning of the ward lounge. It was Vic's turn to sweep the floor while Paul polished it. Vic did not want to sweep the floor. He stated defiantly that he just didn't want to and no one could make him do it. His two-part statement shifted the focus from the floor to the personal struggle in terms of "you can't make me." A struggle ensued over the issue of who was stronger. Both men reached for baseball bats and had to be restrained by staff and group members.

In therapy, Vic was asked why he disliked the job so much. He became annoyed and again tried a diversion about institutions and being "fucked over." For a long time, he was silent. Finally, in exasperation he stated, "I just wouldn't clean up that shit. Man that's a shitty job." Further questioning revealed that the piles of dust, dirt, and wax actually reminded him of fecal material. There was a tense silence as he reluctantly stated this. His face and jaw tightened as he articulated the explanation. It was apparent that he was being flooded with feelings. He paused as if lost in thought. As he spoke, I questioned the reason for the change in his tone and appearance. We began diagramming. During the following discussion, words and phrases were added to the diagram by mutual consent of the group and Vic. Vic substituted his own comments when there was a disagreement. He was given the option of changing any statement in the diagram.

He went on to say, quietly, that he was remembering things. When he was a child, his home was visited by whites on Christmas. They brought charity packages. He remembered their patronizing comments about how nicely the apartment was fixed up: "It was really a *shitty* place, but they were so nice (*sarcastically*) to us poor blacks." He was furious with his father for not having "enough pride" to throw them out. Later, some pipes burst, and sewage flooded the basement. A black plumber came to repair the damage, and Vic tried to stop him from going into the basement. He could not understand how a black man could voluntarily "wade through all that *shit*." The plumber pushed by, explaining it was his job and "the *shit* washed off." (Did

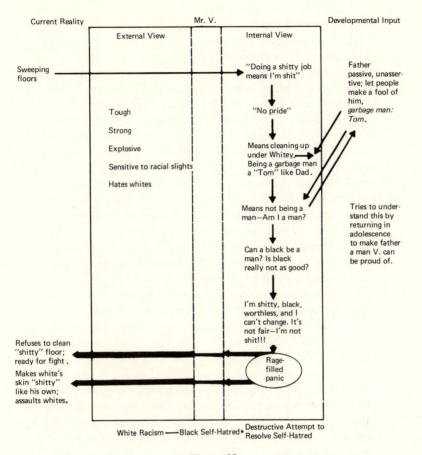

Figure 10

Vic think that there were some things that did not wash off?
See the first internal comment in Figure 10.)

Vic paused and then continued. He remembered
being ashamed of his father for not being more assertive at
home. He could recall times when he was excessively critical of his father as a child and then later in adolescence returning home to try to help his father become more assertive: "Be the man of the house, so I could be proud of
him." His hope had been to create the family structure that
had never existed. When asked why, he could only respond

that for him, something was missing inside. It was as if he couldn't go on in life without one last effort to gain what he had never had in childhood. He described his father in a tearful rage as a passive man, who though strong, let people make a fool of him—"a garbage man, an Uncle Tom." (See description of father in developmental input, Figure 10.)

He then recalled that he had avoided certain sections of town when walking to school in order to avoid seeing his father and acknowledging him in front of his friends. His father was a garbage man and walked behind the truck throwing trash into the truck. Vic said, "He was cleaning up under the white man. I'll never clean up Whitey's *shit!* He was a Tom." (See second section of internal view, Figure 10.) His excessive sensitivity to real or imagined racial slights or questions of manhood made sense in terms of being both black and a man. His fears of being like the father whom he loved began to emerge.

Exploration of a seemingly minor dispute through associative techniques gave valuable insight into Vic's motivation and self-image. He touched upon his own doubts about being a man. All of these issues were succinctly stated with the help of the diagram. By his participating, he could struggle less and make more use of the issues.

Weeks later at a staffing conference, the basic, previously hidden beliefs came to light. Vic had been discussing a time in his life when he had supported himself by brutal assaults. He casually noted as an afterthought that all of his victims had been white. Not only white, but fair-skinned, blond, and blue-eyed. Vic continued to treat this as if it were just an odd coincidence. (See Figure 10, external view and indirect expression of doubts.)

Vic was then asked to describe his actual behavior. It came out that he would pose as a friendly, not too bright black (lame game) and would meet whites in bars. He would then arrange for drugs, women, or gambling. The gullible white would accompany Vic to his apartment. When they were safely inside, a confederate would knock on the door, saying that it was a police raid. Vic would lead the victim out of a back door into an alley. Although armed with a pistol, Vic would pick up a bat and beat the man with it. When asked for details, Vic uncomfortably stated that he always hit the man in the face.

"Where?"

"Man, that's not important."

"No, tell me anyway."

"Shit! I'd hit him in the nose."

"Then?"

"That's all."

"Just the nose?"

Vic glanced about uncomfortably and fidgeted: "Why do we have to discuss this?"

"Because it's important. Just the nose?"

"No, man, I beat 'em up good—the nose, the mouth, the jaw."

The interviewer attempted to ask: Why would he be so foolish as to take the extra time to beat up the man and risk detection, when he could have used his gun and more quietly and quickly robbed him. Angrily, Vic said there was no particular reason, but he agreed it sounded stupid. The interviewer then quietly reviewed the circumstances. For no apparent reason, Vic always chose tall, thin, blond whites. For no apparent reason, he risked detection by beating them. For no apparent reason, the beating usually involved using a bat across the nose, mouth, and jaws. Vic glared at the interviewer silently.

"And, what are you thinking, Vic?"

"I'm just picturing you—there on the ground—your face beat in."

"And what do I look like?" (Already sensing the answer.)

"Your nose is flat, and your cheeks and lips are puffed out and bloody, your teeth on the ground."

Vic paused, his facial expression changing to apparent amazement.

"Who has a flat nose, puffy cheeks and lips?"

Vic paused and did not answer.

"Did you think of that while you were assaulting your victims?"

Quietly, in a trancelike voice and with little awareness of others in the room, he said, "Their skin, their smooth white skin. I made them as shitty and ugly as me!"

Little more needed to be said at that time. In subsequent weeks, we reviewed these episodes and reworked Figure 6.

We explored and found that he believed that being black was being ugly. Later discussion linked this to the view of himself as being shitty by virtue of being black. He was furious at being burdened with the unfair disadvantage that he felt he could never overcome, his skin color.

Clearly, Vic was influenced by the reality of the black status in our society. However, his specific behavior was motivated by an internal perception of himself as being second-rate, shitty, black. He expected all whites automatically to view him as inferior and resented what he really was. As he saw it, he would never even have a chance to prove himself. The man whose murder he had been acquitted of was a white, who had outsmarted him. Vic remembered feeling at that time that he had to erase this person because he was evidence of Vic's inferiority: "He was all those laughing white motherfuckers—if they couldn't respect me, they'd damn well fear me!" (Figure 10, external view).

Vic did not commit himself to drug abstinence during his 6 months in Lexington. He did begin to view whites as individuals, not as a unified group, and became friendly with several. He once related imagining a particular white staff woman as his mother. His hatred greatly diminished. He demonstrated that white racism as it affects the individual can breed black self-hatred and lead to a violent outcome. We cannot devalue a person without everyone's paying the price. This, if for no other reason, makes equality a pragmatic necessity.

Clearly, the kinds of reactions described in these examples do not deal with the underlying problems. They are defensive attempts to deny the issue rather than explore and resolve it. The diagram allows the men to see the basis of their behavior in a concise, understandable manner. Because the diagram develops step by step, its logic remains clear throughout and can be reviewed.

At all times, the men were asked to choose their own words or phrases to describe something. Frequently, they argued over a phrase and its meaning and ultimately chose their own. This is particularly important, because the difference in words is usually minimal, but the use of the man's own words *in writing* committed him in a way that verbal communication would not. The act of acknowledging that a written word or phrase is accurate about you becomes an incontestable issue and ties you to it. We have found that whole patterns of behavior—such as passivity, shyness, extraversion, indecisiveness, and character ridigity—can be understood through the use of this diagrammatic system. The diagramming system can be altered in a flexible manner that adheres to the principles of mutual discussion and collaboration. It is only an aid to understanding; Example 3 shows some of these variations.

Example 3: Claudia was a 17-year-old Caucasian woman who was admitted to the psychiatric service for evaluation following a heroin overdose. She was the eldest of four children and had grown up in a white ghetto. In the psychiatric unit, as she had been throughout her childhood, Claudia was a silent, hostile, friendless, and sullen person. She avoided socializing with the other patients, even during the evenings when there were few staff members around. This was usually the time when even the quietest patients were most active.

Slowly, she gave a history of chronic isolation and withdrawal. When Claudia was five her father began a prison sentence and was never heard from again. A former boxer, he had been a local hero who became the enforcer for a gang. When her father was jailed, Claudia's mother began drinking and no longer took care of the children. Claudia soon became aware that she was poorer and less well cared for than other ghetto residents. Her already injured sense of pride was further diminished when she realized that her mother did not care about Claudia's appearance or hygiene. With angry mortification, she told how the children had teased her one day when a cockroach crawled from her hair. By the end of second grade, she made a conscious effort to avoid people. Repeatedly, she saw a stark contrast between her own pathetic circumstances and the idealized family life portrayed in television, magazines, movies, and schoolbooks.

During her grammar school years, Claudia's mother became a prostitute in order to support the family. Because she frequently brought customers to the apartment, Claudia was repeatedly exposed to displays of brutality, alcoholism, and sexuality. She painfully recalled how she had tearfully covered her head with a pillow in order to shut out the noise and her own sense of powerlessness. She was aware that the men beating and using her mother in the next room were providing the money and food to maintain the household. (The reader might consider what it would be like to realize that one's clothes and food were a result of such pain-filled nights. It is no wonder that children exposed to such home experiences are not able to concentrate quietly in school. Not only do they lack the calm, quiet experiences they also need action and discord to distract them from the painful memories and tumultuous feelings.)

By age 8, Claudia was stealing to supplement the family's income as well as to supply her own needs. Later in her treatment, under group pressure, she revealed that at 11 she had begun a series of incestuous activities with her mother. While this activity was exciting, it conflicted with her wishes for a normal family life. She knew something was wrong. "That's not how a mother is supposed to be." At 13, she left home after a dispute with her mother. Her mother had reneged on a promise to give Claudia her first new dress, the only gift she had ever been promised. Her change of mind was a crushing blow. Shortly after that, Claudia moved in with another woman. Her mother abandoned the younger children, who were assigned to various welfare agencies. She left the city and was not heard from for one year.

Throughout all this time, Claudia became more withdrawn but managed to keep going by denying the personal meaning of all these events. She continued to rely on the hope that some day she would be able to bring her mother and father together; and that they, in turn, would take back the younger children. Bringing the family together, she believed, would make up for the years of deprivation. She was sustained by this unrealistic fantasy of reuniting her family.

When she was 15, Claudia received a surprise visit from her mother who was accompanied by her pimp. Claudia realized that her mother was high on drugs but allowed her to come into her apartment. After a brief and superficial chat, Claudia's mother casually suggested that Claudia go to work for her pimp. She further suggested that Claudia demonstrate some sexual acts with her mother to impress him: "No one could do me like you, baby." Claudia was stunned and became hysterical. Her previous incestuous activities had been distorted into strange but somewhat comforting times of closeness with her mother. The invitation to repeat them, and in public, were too much. Claudia's mother was frightened by the outburst. Claudia said repeatedly "That's not how a mother is supposed to be" as if she were having a dialogue with herself.

That night Claudia got stoned on marijuana and wine, activities which had been only occasional prior to her mother's visit. She went on a steady six-month binge of alcohol and drugs and ended up hooked on heroin. She explained her getting stoned the night of the visit as a result of feeling, "What's the use. It's hopeless. It's like I'm empty inside. There is nothing that will make it better." We diagrammed the situation in two ways, by the familiar rectangle cut by the vertical divider between external and internal (Figures 12A and 12B) and again by a time line connecting the various milestones in her life (Figure 11).

This history was obtained and organized in a series of group and individual sessions. The turning point seemed clear, but why then and not at other times that seemed just as painful? Claudia had been aware of everything outlined before that. Why was the visit the turning point? Figure 7 postulates a continual downhill course, with significant

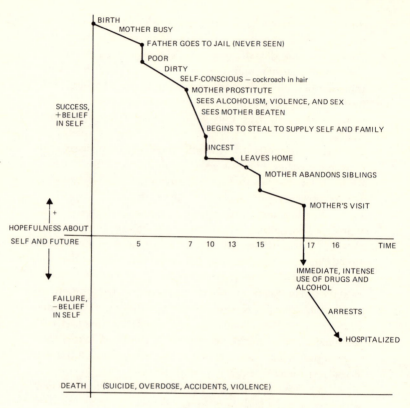

Figure 11

events causing an increased rate of deterioration. As noted, many people with character problems view their life as a continuous decline in which their only role is to try to diminish the inevitable rate of decay. Thus, Claudia could easily agree with the life course shown in Figure 7. The diagram organized the life events from a confusing welter of trauma to an easily discerned series of connected events. Now, the question of why the visit was so significant began to make sense to Claudia. She could understand people's puzzlement. Why didn't the other events cause the flight into drugs?

Having clarified the reason for the question and having

constructed a framework for viewing the course of events in her life, the group began looking for the personal elements. (Involved in all of this was a group process to help support Claudia's participation.)

Claudia, who was initially presented herself as the victim of circumstances, then began speaking of her personal involvement with these situations. She asked: "If she had not left, would her mother not have gone away? Would her brother and sisters be together now?" In reviewing the visit, she changed the words "eat me" to "do me." Why would a person so accustomed to coarse talk be so discreet? The choice of words became a key issue. With hesitancy, anger, and apparent guilt, she revealed the previously concealed incestuous experiences. With great emotion she stated, "It's not supposed to be that way. A mother isn't supposed to be like that. She is supposed to have respect, to be like a mother is supposed to be."

With continued pressure, Claudia spoke of herself as an empty, unwanted, dirty, unneeded, hopeless person. These were written down as her previously denied internal self-image (Figure 12A). With the help of some of these diagrams, she was able to see that she had sustained herself by the unrealistic hope of bringing the family together again. At the time of the visit this changed. Her level of functioning shifted from Figure 12A to Figure 12B. The hope was gone. Her external view of herself had been overwhelmed by the negative beliefs that she had previously denied. Her defenses against the impact of the past events and their implications were shattered. *The drugs had been an attempt to construct a defense against these feelings of hopelessness.* They dulled the pain! (Figure 12B).

Following the therapy meeting in which this became apparent, Claudia did change. She spoke more clearly. She began presenting material about herself and attempting to understand it in terms of her internal perceptions of herself. For the first time, she began seeking out the staff to go over the information. She asked whether it was possible to change. Previously, this question had never arisen. She became energetic. Her appearance and personal hygiene greatly improved. Her work continued for another four

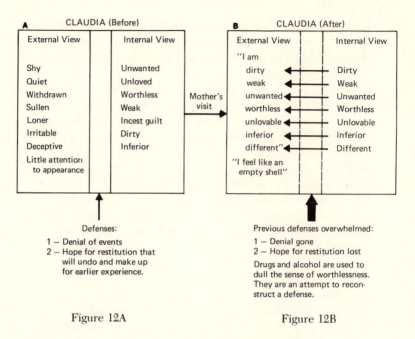

Figure 12A   Figure 12B

years. Although she had many other difficult times, she continued to improve. Frequently, she reflected on the group meetings where these events occurred.

The diagramming technique has proved useful in the treatment of people other than addicts who cannot objectively view their distorted interactions. It has been of use with agitated adolescents who have difficulty in observing the interaction of their emotions and their behavior. Where neurotic patients have used defenses of projections, displacement, and distortion, such diagrams have helped them to view themselves more realistically and to begin the process of therapy. It has helped to reduce the sense that the therapist is judging the patients as harshly as he judges himself.

Another kind of diagram was also employed to help people see the recurrent nature of their life patterns as well as some of the functions of the patterns.

Lonnie was a 34-year-old divorced man, the eldest of nine children. In the hospital he was an articulate, intellectual, and insightful individual who saw others' behavior patterns but not his own. His history was full of promising starts in high school, college, jobs, and marriage. All failed. He began using heroin at age 24, when he was fired from a promising job. His wife left him because of assaultive and irresponsible behavior. Although she was supporting the household, he beat her one day for not having his clothes ironed.

His early life until age 12 was a time of closeness to his mother. She praised his school performance, told him he was special, and admonished him to avoid the coarse and rowdy neighborhood boys. She always warned that failure to listen would result in his becoming a no-good, a thief, and a drunk like his absent father.

At age 12, he tired of being a "mama's boy" and decided to be "independent, a man." He stopped attending church, drank, and skipped school but managed to get through. (His mother was a teacher in an adjacent school.) He entered college on the basis of aptitude tests, interviews, and scholarships for disadvantaged youth (all applied for by his mother). In college, he married a woman who spent much of her time, together with his mother, trying to get him to change. Their methods were bribery in exchange for *promises* of improvement, for example, a new car if he would promise to study and stop drinking and using drugs.

Lonnie was questioned further about his alleged "independence." He was asked about his arrests. Bail, lawyers, and counseling were all arranged for by mother or wife. His mother, like others mentioned, would tell him not to go out or he would be arrested. Indeed, he was. What he called his mother's clairvoyance was easily shown to be something else: a curious lack of caution during some illegal activity, or ignoring a danger signal that he normally would be attuned to. He made his mother's prophecy come true! As he spoke, the following pattern of behavior in Figure 13 emerged.

Complying with her positive wishes meant not being a man—being a Mama's boy. Fulfilling her negative expecta-

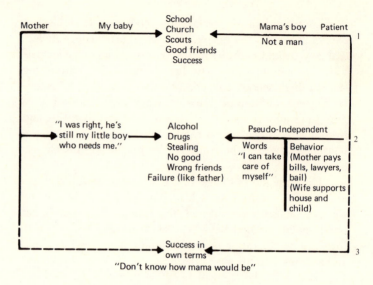

Figure 13

tions did three things: (1) confirmed her belief ("He's still my little boy and needs me to take care of bail, lawyer, etc."), thus maintaining her tie to him; (2) allowed him to act on his anger toward his mother and himself; and (3) enabled him to identify with the man of the family, his father.

For many people, the diagramming system became a first step in allowing them to shift their focus to themselves. It was especially useful with persons who tried to ignore their inner conflicts and stress their external image as viewed by others. It is clearly a device that in itself does not cure or lead to dramatic changes. It does help the individual to begin the therapeutic work of self-observation.

This became clearer for Lonnie when he was asked why he had not been successful on his own terms—as a bookmaker or a numbers man? These are relatively safe illegal activities.

The question of the never developed, successful third option—success or failure on his own terms—upset him. He responded, "I don't know. I'm not sure what she would have done." He was asked what he meant. His answer: "I don't know what she would have done." More discussion revealed that he feared that success would leave him alone when he still felt the need for support. He could not conceive of being different. By being a failure in his mother's terms, Lonnie was assured of ongoing ties to her. He remarked that she sent a sibling to his apartment daily to check up on him, even though he was the eldest. The pattern of maintaining ties by self-destructive behavior can be seen in many addicts whose families support them, frequently helping them to maintain pathology. As with the other diagrams, this provided a useful vehicle for helping a man to see himself as an active participant and not the passive victim in his own life. Arguments and projections stopped. Mutual interest focused on understanding the actual reasons for his actions. He learned his own psychodynamics.

Implicit in all of the foregoing is the premise that effective therapy requires more than mere identification of the problem. A number of people have questioned the necessity of exploring the underlying causes of behavior. They reason that getting a person to see his behavior as self-destructive will automatically lead him to change it. I have never seen this occur. Where there are more serious underlying issues, merely identifying the behavior does not appear to be sufficient to alter it. A steady process of remembering, rethinking, observing, and understanding leads to a general reappraisal of oneself. Anguished memories, distorted beliefs, all must be steadily reworked as old conflicts are resolved.

CHAPTER 8

Treatment

The process of dynamic psychotherapy has been described as being similar to the peeling of an onion. Removing one layer only uncovers another as the process of searching out and understanding progresses. The treatment approaches mentioned thus far indicate a situation in which the metaphor is extended. Here the therapist and the patient must dig up the onion, brush off the soil that distorts its shape, and establish that the onion exists as an entity apart from its surroundings. All of this preparation must occur before the mutual work of carefully uncovering each layer of the personality begins.

Preconceived Distortions

Any treatment situation requires the meeting of two individuals or groups: one is designated as counselor–therapist, and the second is designated as being in need of or seeking help. Each individual or group enters the treatment situation with preconceived views of the other: biases, wishes, doubts, and anxieties. Staff members, for example, tend to categorize from past experience individuals who have chronic and relapsing problems (addicts, criminals, alcoholics, and some psychotic patients). This categorization can be further explained as a sense that one knows and understands a particular individual and that there is little need to observe and plan further. Such pigeonholing allows the staff member to feel certain of his own understanding and thereby reduce any anxiety. Because this is often a mutual process, the patient and the groups involved may collaborate to reassure each other that their original superficial evaluations were accurate and that no further thinking is indicated. The following is an example of the danger of this procedure:

> A 42-year-old mother of five was admitted to an inpatient service for her 12th psychiatric admission in 15 years. She had been previously hospitalized for psychotic episodes in a number of different psychiatric hospitals. She had been treated with varieties of medications and shock treatments and had had batteries of psychological tests.
>
> A medical student had carefully prepared the facts of her life history and hospitalizations and felt he understood the woman. The woman had been raised by rigid and dogmatic parents. She had been sickly and had required special care. Shortly after high school, she had married and moved to a different city. She then began having babies and psychotic episodes. Reports from other hospitals and her current hospital experience indicated that an inability to separate adequately from her own mother coupled with the burdens of raising a large family led to periodic outbursts of abusive behavior and alcoholism. These culminated in psychotic episodes requiring hospitalization.
>
> The student was dissatisfied by several aspects of the situation. After several weeks of hospitalization, the patient seemed composed. She smiled and chatted comfortably with no evidence of psychosis. She denied that her previous behavior during this episode was anything more than a mild upset due to her meddling in-laws. The facts that her husband had filed for divorce and that her children were scattered among her husband's family were ignored by the patient. The student felt that she was impossible to talk with.
>
> The patient's course was similar to that of previous hospitalizations. The ward staff treating the patient viewed her

as chronic and of little interest; they knew her. Her treatment and hospitalization were routine.

The student presented the foregoing material to a group of residents and a senior psychiatrist. His presentation focused upon his vague misgiving that there was something missing in this woman's treatment. Was this all that psychiatry had to offer? The senior psychiatrist asked what the residents understood of her dynamics. There was quick agreement among them that this was a clear case of inadequate separation from an intense relationship with the mother. They were then asked what factors had contributed to her excessive ties and inability to separate. What issue periodically became so painful that this woman became psychotic? To these questions, no one had answers. "You mean, no one has asked her what is so troubling to her that she becomes psychotic?" he said. "She won't talk to us," they replied. Another resident stated that she was chronic and little could be done for her beyond supportive therapy with adjustments in medication and periodic hospitalization.

The patient was asked to join the staff to talk over her situation. She entered the room smiling and chatting. How glad she was to see everyone. She felt so much better. Her manner was superficial but organized. The psychiatrist stated that he was puzzled. He didn't understand what troubled the patient so much that she had recurrent episodes of confusion and disorganization. The patient smiled but rephrased the question and answered as if the trouble were in the past. The psychiatrist twice repeated "problems are," and twice she smilingly stated "problems were."

Their discussion continued, and the interviewer again stated his puzzlement: "I don't know what assures you that you will not experience this again. You don't seem to have understood or dealt with whatever upsets you. Since it has come up so many times in the past and nothing is any clearer now, I assume that the next time you encounter this unknown difficulty, you will become upset again."

The patient's smile disappeared, and she glared at the doctor. Her smile then reappeared, and she discussed various aspects of what he had said. Each time, she responded to comments or questions that were slight alterations of the physician's comments. When he observed that she seemed to want to answer only her version of questions, she began rambling in a confused, psychotic manner. He continued by commenting that something in their interaction seemed to have affected her: Did she understand what it was? She responded psychotically that he could know by talking to all of the previous doctors, especially at a particular hospital. He responded that her comments were unclear. She said, "You wouldn't want to know what's inside me. All of you doctors. You just ask your questions to get your information. Well, they know at that hospital." Had she told them? "Yes, I told them good." She described an angry outburst at her previous hospital. "Yes," the physician commented, "it appears that anger is a disorganizing experience for you."

"You should only know. It's like a knot inside. It builds up like I'm going to explode."

"And this knot?"

"It strangles my heart like I'm going to die. I can't stand it. It hurts too much."

In a nonpsychotic way, she spoke with alternating anger and sadness. Gradually, she related that her first psychotic episode occurred while she was in high school. Her family disapproved of her boyfriend and insisted that she give him up. Torn between her strong ties with her family and her love for him, she complied with their wishes: "I felt like I was choking. My heart broke."

An emotional bargain was made between the patient and her family. She would comply obediently with their wishes, and they would protect her from the pain of separation and growth. She married a man whom her parents selected. Her periodic psychosis related to unresolved longings for her first love and unresolved rage at her parents for not fulfilling their part of the bargain. She remained in therapy for the next 3 years with a resident who was present at the training conference. During that time, she examined her own needs to remain with her family and the fears of her own emotions. During the course of treatment, she had two psychotic episodes related to the treatment experience. Her need for medication diminished to an occasional sedative at bedtime. It has been 5 years since her last hospitalization.

Had it not been for an inquisitive medical student, this patient and the group of doctors present at that conference might not have seen that treatment requires more than the cataloging of facts. It requires that the therapist and the patient come to understand the origin of the pain that generates destructive behavior.

In this situation, the resident was biased. He was told upon admission that she was a chronic, relatively uninteresting patient whose dynamics were understood. Because that is what he expected to see, that is what he saw.

The patient likewise had seen many psychiatrists who were interested in a historical sequence of facts. Her experiences with these doctors had been of little use. Thus, she entered the conference expecting a futile review of her life circumstances. She was willing to play out the charade: "You ask a question; I'll give a minimal answer. You'll get your teaching done and I'll finish my hospitalization, for a while." Prior to the interview, the patient anticipated that she had little to gain in the conference.

For the process of treatment to begin, the therapist and the patient need to divest themselves of their preconceived views of each other. This is particularly important with impulsive people. They have an exaggerated need to place people in known categories. This process allows them to ignore painful issues or confrontations. An individual is able to attribute questions and comments to the therapist's training, background, etc., and pass over the fact that the questions come from the therapist's experience with him. This shunting aside is seen in comments like: "You people (grouping) always ask questions like that." "Those may be important questions for someone with your training." "Psychiatrists always say things like that!"

Many times, these patients sense the expectations of the therapist and fulfill them. This process is usually automatic and allows the patient to get by with minimal disruption of his pre-

cariously balanced sense of self. Since his goal is frequently compliance in order to gain some other end, one needs to attract his
attention to the treatment situation as a unique experience in
which preconceived stereotypes may not hold.

Gaining the Patient's Attention

During initial interviews, many impulsive people respond
with answers that sound empty and practiced. Although the data
may be accurate, they are given in a bored, unenthusiastic manner. It is as if the person has been over the same material
hundreds of times. He could care less! It has never done him
any good.

At other times, the individual may slouch in his seat or, al-
ternatively, may energetically pursue each question with great
interest. One man answered every question but could not stop
talking or moving about. He was like a frisky puppy in his attempts to be pleasing. His behavior was inconsistent with the
gravity of the issues discussed. Smilingly, he described early
losses and separations. Often, it is such a discrepancy between
the spoken words and the manner of delivery that provides an
opportunity to gain the patient's attention.

The man who had the puppylike quality was told that the
interviewer was puzzled by the discrepancy between his light-
hearted manner and the gravity of the issues he was discussing.
The patient responded that he always smiled and was called
"high tension." He tried to dismiss these observations in order
to continue his well-rehearsed history. The interviewer acknowledged the potential importance of the information but returned
to the puzzling discrepancy. At first, the patient responded as if
these reflections were a criticism. Everybody else accepted the
smiling and constant activity, why couldn't this person? The patient stopped looking around the room and focused his gaze on
the doctor. He was finding the interview distressing and became
more wary.

The psychiatrist began questioning the onset of this high

tension quality and smiling behavior. Was it recent or lifelong? When did it start? What purpose might it serve? The patient began commenting with "Maybe," "Probably," and "I guess." Again, the psychiatrist interrupted, saying that he needed to guess because he did not know the answers but that the patient merely had to slow down and look inside: "But when I do that, I just stop. Then I get depressed and need the drugs to start up." Further discussion uncovered episodes in which this sequence of slowing down was in fact followed by depression and drug abuse. At other times, the depression was followed by violent behavior and a return of the hyper quality. All of the episodes of slowing down followed losses: a death, parental divorce, and failure to finish a tour of duty in the service.

Observing discrepancies in behavior, manner, and verbal content—whether they be manifested by boredom, practiced speeches, inappropriate joking, excessive friendliness, or hostility—lets the patient know that the therapist is attentive and interested. Presenting these observations in a firm, clear manner that is nonpunitive—neutral—may startle the patient. *It is crucial that the therapist make his clarification of issues in a straightforward manner devoid of personal rancor. Thus, the observations stand apart from whatever feeling the therapist and the patient have for each other. This allows the observation to be defined as an issue for the patient to work on and understand.*

Focusing upon behavior can cause the patient to become increasingly anxious. In the preceding example, the patient became wary and began staring only at the therapist. His anxiety made him more aware of the therapist and caused him to pay attention. He later reflected that he "hadn't been sure what to expect." The anxiety became productive as he could no longer take the interviewer for granted. His previous experience with interviews led him to expect that he could get by with a historical review and a few clichés, and that would be all. The *intrusive* observations made him more watchful and more thoughtful.

In other situations, patients may consistently avoid looking at the therapist. As with other behavior, it is helpful to try and understand the meaning of the failure to look at the interviewer.

Sometimes it is many months before one understands this issue. At other times, its meaning is clear almost immediately. I have seen a number of patients in whom the avoidance of eye contact came to indicate shame, low self-esteem, or the fear that the interviewer would read their thoughts. Sometimes it is a means of blocking out the reality of the therapist's existence and the reality of their discussion. When this occurs the therapist may ask the patient to look at him in order to help him concentrate upon what they are saying.

Whatever the situation, the therapist and the patient need to be certain that they have each other's attention. If not, then a useless charade may ensue.

Structure, Limits, Goals

Any life situation has its structure, limits, and goals. The previous chapters emphasize these factors in treatment. While treatment of more neurotic patients usually has some explicit structure and limits, there are usually a number of shared implicit limits. Therapist and patient expect defined treatment times and fees. They work out arrangements for vacations and emergency contact. Implicit is the mutual understanding that there is to be no physical intimacy or violence. It is understood that the therapist is available only on a limited basis and cannot be a substitute for people and relationships in the patient's life. The patient enters treatment with the view that he is suffering from distress, even if its nature is unclear. The goal of treatment is the clarification and resolution of the problem.

The impulsive person has few of these understandings when he enters therapy. Once the individual's pretherapy expectations are clarified and his attention is gained, he needs to define his own goals. The therapist may need to be extremely active at this point. A basically depressed and hopeless person does not have many goals. Therefore, limited goals may initially include an understanding of discrepancies in behavior that occur in the interview setting. Successful clarification gives the patient a small example of the process of treatment. Frequently, this engenders some hope that leads to the development of goals.

It is well to review problems of violence, sexuality, intimacy, drug use, medications, and confidentiality at the outset.

Example: Mona is a 32-year-old executive secretary for a large law firm. Her employer had called the therapist that morning to request an appointment for Mona that day. She came to the appointment accompanied by her roommate, who had watched her on the previous night to keep her from killing herself. In spite of her excellent work record at a complex job, she felt worthless. She had been drinking and using Demerol nightly for years. Periodically, she had become suicidal and made secret attempts. Her manner was direct, clear, and businesslike. She was going to kill herself. What was the therapist going to do to stop her? The therapist responded that her request had been for therapy. How did a threat of suicide show an interest in therapy? Therapy had the goal of problem solving. Suicide was a solution that precluded therapy. If she merely wanted someone to protect her from suicide, she could try a hospital. He further clarified that hospitalization was no guarantee of such protection, since people committed suicide in hospitals. If she was interested in therapy, they had something to discuss. She was shocked by his response. Didn't he understand her desperation? "No," he responded. She had only told him that she was going to commit suicide and then told him it was his responsibility. She had not discussed her desperation. He was merely informing her that her request for him to assume responsibility for her was impossible for him to comply with and not part of therapy. Therapy required her to be responsible for keeping herself alive and for discussing without action her problems and needs. The patient could not believe that the doctor would not comply with her stated needs. Again, he explained the requirements of therapy and their inconsistency with her initial request. She burst out laughing and said that no one ever dared to speak to her that way.

The two then settled down to review her situation. Her many achievements had not diminished an intense self-

hatred and driving pressure to justify her existence. The
therapist listened and questioned further until they both
were clear about the several painful losses that she had experienced. The therapist shifted from his more rigorous initial demeanor and empathetically acknowledged the pain
that Mona was experiencing. She seemed comforted by this
and supported by the therapist's understanding. He questioned whether she had ever reviewed this issue with other
therapists and what had been the outcome.

Indeed, she had seen four previous therapists. All
were competent individuals. The patient and two of the
previous therapists had found that opening these emotion-
laden areas led to the outpouring of a torrent of unmanagea-
ble feeling. The patient became disorganized with these
emotions and suicidal.

Although a review and understanding of these issues
seemed necessary, the process could be destructive. In
order to guard against this, the patient and the therapist
agreed that the patient needed more solid "anchors in reality" before they could begin investigating these highly
charged areas. These anchors included stable relationships
with people, regular work hours, diminished alcohol and
Demerol use, and observing and stopping particular impulsive responses. Each of these initial goals required months
of review and work. While they ostensibly laid the groundwork for the later "insight work" that she desired, the process of achieving the initial goals taught her a great deal
about her processes of judgment, evaluation, choice, and
decision making.

Another part of the initial agreement was on the use of
behavior versus discussion to communicate distress. The
patient had free access to the therapist's home phone, only
for bona fide emergencies. In addition, she could be admitted to the therapist's private hospital if she asked for help
prior to self-destructive behavior. A request made before
such behavior would indicate a desire to try to work in therapy. Hospitalization after a self-destructive episode would
be at the custodial state hospital, as such actions indicated a
resistance to therapy work. After one stay at each hospital,
the patient realized that her work could not be shortcut by

some magical treatment at a hospital. Indeed, both she and her therapist agreed that hospitalizations interrupted her process of therapy.

Thus, in first interviews she was able to clarify distorted expectations, obtain some sense of short- and long-term goals, and develop an agreement for treatment.

She remained in treatment, and her therapist reports consistent improvement with transient relapses. There have been no suicide attempts in 2 years, and her multiple drug abuse is almost zero.

The four elements of her initial treatment process were (1) firm and gentle clarification of treatment realities and limits; (2) acknowledgment of the therapist's capacity for empathic awareness with the patient; (3) the need to construct a foundation in reality of situations and relationships that would allow the toleration of emotion-laden insight therapy; and (4) the investigation of past events in order to understand their effect upon her present life and her view of herself. The recovery of memories and their associated feelings is a crucial aspect of the treatment process. The early loss and its anguish need to be remembered in order to be validated as genuine. Subsequently, the early primitive interpretation of this loss needs to be uncovered. The ideas that the individual was the cause of the loss and is therefore bad and unlovable require scrutiny. Frequently, there is a turning point in treatment as the patient painfully realizes that the parent never had all that the patient desired. These four steps are often necessary in the development of therapy with impulsive people.

Transference–Countertransference

These two terms relate to the reexperiencing in therapy of emotions, conflicts, and situations that occurred earlier in one's life. Such experiences on the part of the patient are called *transference*. The patient is expected to use this experience in transference as a means to understand and resolve earlier situations that continue to be relived in the present. Thus, a patient may

see the therapist as a most understanding, thoughtful, trustwor-
thy person. Such a perspective may be out of proportion to the
reality of the experience of therapist and patient together and
may indicate some yet-to-be-clarified doubt, wish, need, etc.
Similarly, a patient may be seductive with a therapist and wish
for an intimate relationship. Again, this behavior needs to be investigated and understood. Other emotions, such as disproportionate rage and criticism of the therapist, likewise need the
same process of reality testing and investigation.

The therapist who is seduced into sexual or angry relationships with his patients is dealing with his own needs and
unresolved conflicts (countertransference). Thus, it is necessary
for therapists to understand their own drives and motivations.
Such understanding helps them to be more effective in the primary task of assisting their patients. In spite of claims to the contrary, the radical therapies that support intimate relationships of
patient and therapist seem to be an excuse for therapists to in-
dulge their own fantasies and unresolved problems.

The pressures upon therapists in the area of transference
and countertransference are very high in work with impulsive
people. Their initial demands for immediate gratification or
proof of the therapist's value shift to a constant testing of the
relationship. Because an impulsive person's needs are so great
and his previous experience with consistency is minimal, he cannot believe that the therapist will do what he says. Therefore, he
constantly looks for evidence of deception or diminished interest. If he can prove that the therapist is like every other disappointing person, he is less upset by his early life losses. Should
the therapist prove to be different, the patient must face the
contrast between the therapist's availability and the parental
unavailability. This contrast increases his distress and anxiety in
treatment. Thus, the patient has conflicting wishes for the therapist. On the one hand, he wants a thoughtful, consistent therapist; on the other, there is a wish for a disappointing individual.

The absence of significant, successful previous life experiences coupled with the lack of any real concept of the impulsive

person's own role in treatment further exacerbates the pressure upon the therapist.

Many beginning therapists find themselves alternately excited, angry, bored, fatigued, and depressed by their work. They seem to share the same emotional swings as their patients. Frequently, they feel alone and different from others in the field. Many quit or conclude that the task is hopeless. Those working with addicts may opt for drug maintenance with little hope of change.

Several supports are necessary to help these therapists: (1) regular staff meetings at which staff problems are reviewed and worked out; (2) case supervision; (3) teaching by senior therapists; (4) demonstration interviews or videotapes; and (5) an active private life separate from the treatment setting. The first four items introduce a perspective that diminishes the sense of isolation. The fifth item is extremely important. Many young therapists immerse themselves in the treatment program and develop their social relationships within the staff. Their work and their social life involve the same people. They come to identify themselves and their self-esteem totally with the work. Dissatisfaction and disappointment in one area are not counterbalanced by positive experiences in the other.

"Different Strokes for Different Folks"

Not all impulsive people require or respond to the same treatment methods. This is particularly true early in treatment. Those impulsive people who abuse substances may require detoxification and physical rehabilitation before they are able to enter any more psychological treatment.

Alcohol

In some ways alcohol is the most dangerous and difficult abuse substance to deal with. Its wide use and availability are compounded by the capacity for insidious physical deterioration and dependency. After the initial detoxification, involvement in Alcoholics Anonymous with or without a supportive living environment is necessary. Alcoholics Anonymous provides many needed supports that usual therapies lack. These include an individual sponsor—the person who helps the alcoholic get to the meetings and supports his involvement. There is 24-hour support and availability. Daily group meetings with other people like the alcoholic who are in various stages of reconstitution give clear examples of the possibility of change. There is a structured program for change. This is linked to both an explanation of his disease—that the individual has an inherent incapacity to handle alcohol and will never be able to tolerate its use—and a belief in a higher ethical and universal power (God). There is no guilt or criticism. The patient is just allergic to alcohol; that's the way he was created. The ultimate steps of the program allow an individual to give the kind of help he initially received. This process of helping others reinforces the renewed sense of self-dignity. While I do not accept the belief system of AA, I respect the process and the usefulness of its system of help.

Because of the physiological and emotional effects of alcohol upon the individual, many therapists believe that any form of psychotherapy is useless unless the patient has been free of alcohol and in AA for at least a year. My experience with alcoholism is limited, but I have seen instances in which this is true and other instances in which psychotherapy was both useful and necessary concurrent with detoxification and AA. It seems to be true that some subtle thought processes do not reconstitute for months after the initial detoxification.

Some individuals believe that Alcoholics Anonymous is the only necessary treatment and that all others are superfluous. Again, my experience is limited to a number of patients and acquaintances of whom this is not true. The energies that were consumed in the destructive period of alcoholism may now be turned into excessive compensation through work or scrupulous attention to family or AA. For some people, the constant involvement in AA does seem an adequate substitute for the losses postulated in Chapter 4. In order for it to work, however, they must maintain a consistent involvement. Without some understanding and resolution of the early sequence of loss followed by guilt at a time of developing impulse control, the individual does not grow beyond the need for compensation for the loss. Those former alcoholics who become model family men and excessively committed to their work or to benevolent projects frequently display the same consuming drive that was present during their period of alcohol abuse. The compensatory behavior can be a new attempt to deal with the personal sense of worthlessness. From alcoholics, they have become workaholics.

Sedative–Hypnotic Addiction

Addiction to sedative medications requires careful detoxification because of the hazards of seizures and death. Following the initial 1–2 weeks of withdrawal, the individual may continue to display irritability, poor appetite, and sleep disturbances for several weeks or months. When this occurs, it is not clear whether this is a period of readjustment of biological rhythms, a reemergence of psychological problems that the medication masked, or a more subtle, prolonged, direct effect of substance abuse.

Addiction to sedative–hypnotics, unlike the addiction to alcohol, requires the individual to become involved in either illegal means of procurement or deception of physicians and druggists to maintain an adequate supply. The person addicted to sedative–hypnotics, either in response to his addiction or as a result of preaddiction characterologic differences, frequently displays different behavior than that of the alcoholic. Both may be impulsive and aggressive while showing evidence of depression and apathy. People addicted to sedative–hypnotics may shift about in a quest for a drug that more adequately diminishes their sense of dysphoria. Their patterns of abuse may be less stable than those of alcoholics. Many of them are younger people whose searching about may also be a function of their age.

Few programs are geared specifically to the treatment of

people addicted to sedative hypnotics. I have had limited experience with these people but have found characteristics similar to
those of other addicted individuals. During weekly consultations
to a combination inpatient and outpatient program specifically
established for people addicted to multiple drugs, I usually encounter people who relate their addiction to an underlying sense
of worthlessness.

During an interview just prior to this book's completion, I
saw a 26-year-old man with a history of 35 arrests. The following
dialogue ensued:

> Doctor: "I'm puzzled, I don't understand how your life
> got to be such a mess."
> Patient: "I just like getting high on barbs."
> "Just like getting high?"
> "Yeah, it's better than being the way I am."
> "And how is that?"
> "Nothing man—just nothing."
> In short order he shifted from being angry and provok-
> ing to a tearful declaration of his own worthlessness. When
> asked if he had ever felt any different about himself, he
> began reviewing his life and saw a time of change. As the
> reader would expect, there were two losses. One occurred
> during the age period of 3–7 years and the second during
> adolescence.

My experience with such people has led me to believe that
people addicted to sedative–hypnotics are more amenable to
direct psychotherapies after detoxification. These drugs seem to
have less of the disorganizing qualities of alcohol addiction. The
important factor seems to be the willingness of the therapist, the
group, or the treatment center to serve multiple roles from detoxification to more formal therapies. These include the interest
and capacity to help the individual learn to structure his chaotic
life while paying attention to his need for genuine human contact. Such contact, again, includes the necessity of sharing and
reviewing the painful life experiences.

Opiates

Much of the book has dealt with my views of individuals addicted to opiate drugs. Detoxification from these substances is painful but does not contain the risk of seizures and death inherent in alcohol and sedative–hypnotic medication withdrawal. The period of physiological and emotional readjustment seems to be less than that involved in alcohol and sedative–hypnotic addiction.

One difference in the selection of opiates in preference to alcohol and barbiturates may be its capacity to inhibit or diminish rage. Intoxication with alcohol can lead to outbursts of rage, the so-called "nasty drunk" who becomes argumentative and fights. This does not occur while one is intoxicated with opiates. This is also supported by the experience of the individuals mentioned previously, who consciously switched from alcohol to opiates because they feared their violent outbursts while drinking.

This selection difference refers only to the intoxicated state. Withdrawal from any depressant of the central nervous system can lead to irritable, angry, and impulsive behavior.

Treatment Modalities

While I prefer a treatment regimen that includes an investigative process, there are a number of methods or combinations that may be useful. The techniques demonstrated thus far include elements of dynamic psychotherapy of both individual and group varieties, milieu therapy, reality therapy, transactional analysis, confrontation techniques, ego-oriented rational therapies, etc.

More important than the specific modality is the thoughtfulness and sensitivity of the individuals involved in the treatment process. Thus, confrontation techniques may be useful when carefully planned and conducted to meet the individual's needs. Frequently, the style of a method is learned without the understanding of its specific usefulness and limitations. In the early 1970s, confrontation was a much-touted process. In many treatment settings, I saw people humiliated and degraded in loud, abusive harangues called confrontation therapy. The groups had little understanding of the technique. They did it because it was supposed to be "therapeutic."

There was a similar emphasis upon self-help and metha-done programs. Both modalities have genuine potential value. Self-help programs can provide group support and under-standing while giving realistic input about behavior and atti-tudes. Yet, I have seen instances in which the self-help units de-veloped into cults of young people who viewed the outside world as the enemy. Thus, anyone who wanted to leave the set-ting was reviled as a traitor and expelled. How did such resis-tance to separation help an individual who was struggling with growth and separation issues? Whereas Alcoholics Anonymous defines the problem as a personal inability of the individual to tolerate alcohol, some of these self-help programs defined the problem as lying in the so-called bad outside environment or bad society that provided the "bad" drug. Does this help a per-son who is already unable to see his own role in creating his problems?

Methadone as an agent of detoxification can ease the dis-comfort and allow early involvement in normal life activities. Chronic methadone maintenance without concomitant treatment does not resolve the underlying problems. Repeatedly, I have seen men maintain themselves on methadone while they at-tempt to rebuild their lives. Outwardly, there were steady im-provements in work, home, and social lives. Careful attention usually demonstrated a continuation of the same process of poor thinking and decision making, difficulty with intimacy, and im-pulsive attempts to use "shortcuts" in achieving goals while on methadone. After a year or two of visible gains, the individual frequently requested detoxification from methadone because he was "better." He had a job and an allegedly stable home life and was going to school. After 6 months or a year, he would be back requesting methadone maintenance. While some colleagues would respond that such a request is evidence of the chronic and relapsing nature of the illness, I would see it as more directly related to superficial changes that did not touch the underlying personality problem. The individual had continued to function in a characteristic manner while on methadone. No one paid attention to the manner in which he related to school, work, or family.

Clinics that provide methadone in combination with people-oriented therapies have the potential to help the individual make realistic gains in his home and work life. At the same time, they can address the underlying roots of the characterologic distress.

The problem does not seem to be the particular modality of treatment used as much as interest on the part of the therapist and his awareness that more than superficial change is required. The process of uncovering painful losses, deficits, and conflicts and understanding their implications can be accomplished with words, diagrams, psychodrama, or psychoanalysis. The type of treatment must meet the needs of the individual's underlying problems and current capacities for particular kinds of therapy. Therapies that tie together the past experiences with present behavior enhance the individual's capacity to understand himself.

The addicted person has little experience with helpful and satisfying human relationships. Not liking himself, he cannot genuinely become close and intimate with others. The emotional emptiness is transiently relieved by the intoxication or the destructive behavior. This uneasy truce can be relieved only by carefully understood, new human relationships.

These human relationships, while considering the needs of both parties, must deal with the reality of the mutual effects of behavior. The counselor is aware of his own needs and responses. He endeavors to assist his client to consider his own needs and the effects of his behavior. Together they assess and confront the clients life events and his responses to them, both current and past. Decisions, judgments, and consequences are reviewed. Personal beliefs are elucidated and investigated. This process, with its constant need for realistic input, is a task requiring years of consistency. During this process, the individual with the impulsive character can change and become less troubled, so long as he is *never* humiliated or degraded in the process.

Conclusion

In this book I have described various symptoms of impulsive behavior as responses to a common underlying character defect. This defect develops in childhood when maternal support is removed by death, physical illness, or emotional withdrawal. Without adequate recognition of and substitution for this loss, the individual continues to develop in some areas but remains arrested in others. A sense of panic and self-devaluation develops. This is reexperienced throughout the individual's life and leads to self-destructive, meaningless violence. In the process of treatment, this loss is identified and validated, but the child's early interpretations of responsibility and inherent lack of lovability are questioned. Such questions can be explored only in another human relationship that pays attention to these early losses and does not attempt to minimize them. It becomes an experience in relearning about the self.

This process takes many years of consistent effort. It is difficult to conceive of its occurring in a society in which divorce is increasing and extended families disintegrating and in which religious and moral values are practiced with duplicity. The very nature of our society—with its penchant for rapid change, unrealistic expectations, and overvaluing of external achievement at the expense of human values—supports the development of character problems.

If people genuinely believed in the espoused principles of our society, one could focus more upon long-range, multigenerational needs. Does anyone believe that people raised in emotional and economic privation are going to support a system that promised a dream and gave nothing? Unfortunately, there is a polarization away from the ineffective programs of social change toward ineffective repression.

I do not advocate massive social-welfare programs that expect dramatic change in a few years. Giving handouts of food, money, or meaningless jobs is stupid and insulting to a recipient. Most people want and need an opportunity to develop their own skills by hard work. They do need opportunities and support for this process to occur.

Our increasing problems with impulsive behavior, violence, drug abuse, and family dissolution will continue. What is needed is a national long-term planning and evaluation process that will help reorient our society to focus upon the process of family and community development. Hopefully, a system of ethics will develop with a realistic sense of shared responsibility for oneself, one's family, and one's community. At the same time, the problems of the millions of casualties of our mindless social climate must be heeded. The millions of alcoholics, criminals, addicts, etc., will not go away. They continue to live and re-create the same problems that spawned them. Whereas Moses could spend 40 years in the desert waiting for the older generation of slaves to die off, we have no such option. The same kind of effort that mobilized the country in wartime is necessary if we are to begin to understand our spreading malignancy. Such an effort will require not years of work but generations.

Index

"Confrontation avoidance" game,
  125-126
Conscience
  guilt and, 90-91
  punishment from, 47
Consciousness level, games and, 96
"Contracts" game, 102-103
Counseling, discomfort in, 50
Counselor, in games program, 97-98
Countertransference, in treatment,
  191-193
Crime, drug addiction and, 31-32
Criticism, inability to handle, 56-57

Denial, violence and, 146
Depression, 40-67
  acting out of, 70
  anxiety or discomfort in, 61-62
  avoidance of feeling in, 52-54
  avoidance techniques in, 48-49
  discontinuity of events in, 55-56
  emotional loss and, 78
  entitlement in, 59-61
  examples of, 67-70
  inability to accept criticism in, 56-
    57
  inability to delay gratification in,
    58-59
  inability to form close personal
    relationships in, 41-44
  inability to plan in, 57-58
  low self-esteem in, 40-41
  manipulation in, 44-48
  parental abandonment and, 80-81
  self-destruction in, 63-70
  self-evaluation failure in, 49-52
  "unreal people" in, 54-55
Destructive behavior, outside of
  treatment, 142-144, see also
  Violence
Destructive personality disorder, 37-
  38
Detoxification, listlessness following,
  69
Development, normal, 72-75
Developmental defect, 71-93
Diagnostic and Statistical Manual,
  38

Discomfort, inability to suffer, 61-
  62
"Distractions" game, 107-108
"Do as I Say" game, 128-129
Drives, doubts about, 78-79
Drug abuse, 4, see also Drug addict;
  Drug addiction
  character problems and, 6
  outpatient clinic for, 35-36
Drug addict
  alcoholism in background of, 29
  anger of toward "connected" person,
    65
  basic beliefs of, 32
  black/white ratio in, 31
  character change and, 1
  chemical and biological changes
    in, 88
  composite patient as, 29-32
  crime record of, 31-32
  denial and, 21-22
  depression and, see Depression
  economic background of, 29-30
  emotional loss and, 75-76
  father role in adolescence of, 30-
    31
  game behavior in, 18-19
  guilt in, 78
  hopelessness of, 14-15, 20-21
  as "human beings," 24
  impulsive character pathology of,
    xvii
  incest and, 76-77
  most pronounced current symptom
    in, 10
  mother role in, 20
  at "Narco," see National Institute
    of Mental Health
  premises about, 10-22
  rewards and freedom for, 18
  rule violations by, 16
  "single type" of, 11 n.
  treatment paradox for, 21-22
  treatment programs for, 17
  violence in character structure of,
    144
Drug addiction
  case history of, 8-9